Interpreting Health Benefits and Risks

Erik Rifkin • Andrew Lazris

Interpreting Health Benefits and Risks

A Practical Guide to Facilitate
Doctor-Patient Communication

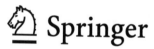 Springer

Erik Rifkin
Rifkin and Associates
Baltimore, MD, USA

Andrew Lazris
St. Agnes Hospital
Baltimore, MD, USA

ISBN 978-3-319-11543-6   ISBN 978-3-319-11544-3 (eBook)
DOI 10.1007/978-3-319-11544-3
Springer Cham Heidelberg New York Dordrecht London

Library of Congress Control Number: 2014951362

Printed on acid-free paper

Springer is part of Springer Science+Business Media (www.springer.com)

To Scott and Jason
Very good friends who also happen
to be my sons

E. Rifkin

To my beautiful wife Cathy, the love of my
life, and to my amazing kids Michael, David,
and Rachel

A. Lazris

Foreword

"Doctor" comes from classical Latin "teacher, adviser". (It is also related, more distantly, to "decent".) In modern medicine the role of teacher has reassumed prominence in the work of doctors. The idealized paradigm now is shared decision-making; doctors provide real, accurate information (teach), help patients articulate goals, and advise on strategies to achieve these goals. The patient decides.

As is often the case with paradigms, reality is a bit sloppier than this. The shenanigans of Big Pharma and the device makers and the lurking threat of litigation are in the exam room when doctor and patient talk. The doctor's desire to get paid may intrude. The vagaries of human decision-making are there too. Osler said that the main thing that distinguishes man from the animals is the desire to take medication. The contemporary yearning for risk-free existence dovetails with the ancient, widespread and deeply held desire not to be dead. In the exam room, the balance tilts strongly towards doing something. Overtreatment is ascendant.

How does good doctoring create meaningful shared decision-making and limit overtreatment? You will see in the pages of this book. Andrew Lazris is a seasoned, thoughtful clinician who has obviously spent a lot of time thinking about how to teach his patients. He is also an unbiased, careful reader of the medical literature. Erik Rifkin is an environmental scientist with decades of experience teaching individuals and organizations about risk evaluation with respect to environmental threats. Together they have written *Interpreting Health Benefits and Risks: A Practical Guide to Facilitate Doctor-Patient Communication*, in which they provide the essential ingredients to help patients make sensible decisions in a world that will always be risky.

The book considers several high-stakes decisions that are likely to be familiar to readers. Should I get a mammogram? A blood test for prostate cancer? Should I take a statin? An aspirin? What about antibiotics for sinusitis? Blood thinners to prevent stroke in atrial fibrillation? And many other treatment decisions that doctors and patients are making every day. For each, precise, referenced data about the benefits and risks associated with the intervention are presented. This is one of the strong points of the book.

A second strong point is the Benefit Risk Characterization Theater. The authors spend some time demonstrating how presenting data as relative risk reduction is routinely misleading; the vaunted 50 % reduction in stroke among people with atrial fibrillation who take Coumadin blood thinner compared to aspirin turns out to be a reduction of not quite one disabling stroke per year. BRCT graphic is the ideal way to grasp this idea more firmly. Their unique visual approach also makes clear just what it means to say, for example, that spiral CT scanning 1,000 patients for lung cancer saves three lives in 5 years, but with a lot of unnecessary and harmful treatment in the group that was screened.

In summary, this book considers several common and important situations where faulty decision-making makes overtreatment a serious risk. Clear, fair, referenced, and useful information is provided. And a powerful intuitive technique is introduced which allows patient and doctor to talk as equals as they work together in the exam room. The authors emphasize that some patients who have been fully educated will still accept high risks of harm for a small chance of avoiding premature death. But as this book is accepted and its ideas and technique are extended, I feel sure that net harm to patients will be curtailed. And what is more, the integrity of the decision-making process will be improved.

Professor of Medicine   Thomas Finucane, MD
Division of Gerontology and Geriatric Medicine
The Johns Hopkins University School of Medicine
Baltimore, MD, USA

Preface

Recently, there has been a dramatic increase in the level of interest and involvement, by private and public institutions, in programs and projects associated with patient-centered care. In light of this significant change in the landscape, we have been motivated to write, *Interpreting Health Benefits and Risks: A Practical Guide to Facilitate Doctor-Patient Communication*. We believe this book to be timely and of value to those supportive of shared decision making (SDM).

There is considerably more awareness today of the need for doctor/patient collaboration than there was just a few years ago. This is due, in part, to the passage of the Affordable Care Act (ACA). ACA has a number of provisions which are designed to address concerns caregivers and patients face when making critical health care choices without key information that would help them make better decisions.

The ACA established the Patient-Centered Outcomes Research Institute (PCORI)—a nonprofit, nongovernmental organization tasked with researching the effectiveness of medical treatments, along with associated risks and benefits. PCORI intends to "help people make informed health care decisions, and improve health care delivery and outcomes, by producing and promoting high integrity, evidence-based information that comes from research guided by patients, caregivers and the broader health care community."

Other well-known public and private organizations have also become involved with initiatives that encourage physicians, patients, and other health care stakeholders to think and talk about medical tests and procedures that may be unnecessary, and in some instances cause harm. For example, *Consumer Reports* is developing and disseminating materials for patients through large consumer groups. Apparently, more than 50 specialty societies have now joined the campaign and over 30 societies will announce new lists in 2014.

The primary purpose of this book will be to make physicians and others in the public health community aware of a unique decision aid designed to improve SDM and empower patients to communicate with their doctors regarding which tests and other medical procedures are right for them. We call this tool a Benefit/Risk

Characterization Theater (BRCT), first introduced in the book, *The Illusion of Certainty; Health Benefits and Risks* (published by Springer in 2007).

The BRCT is a simple, straightforward graphic which presents a clear and objective picture of health benefits and risks associated with specific screening tests, drugs, surgeries, and other types of medical intervention. Subsequent to the release of *The Illusion of Certainty*, we have had many opportunities to utilize BRCTs when communicating with patients regarding forms of medical intervention. Based on our experience using this approach, we are confident that it will help physicians and patients make appropriate decisions together. In fact, a key motivating factor for writing this book is that we now have evidence that our approach works.

A goal of this book is to add a unique dimension to and supplement existing programs and projects which focus on communicating results from comparative effectiveness research, evidence-based medicine, and other efforts to increase meaningful patient-centered care.

Interpreting Health Benefits and Risks: A Practical Guide to Facilitate Doctor Patient Communication is an interdisciplinary book which we believe will be of interest to physicians, patients, nurses, public health organizations, colleges, universities, pharmaceutical companies, professional schools, policy-makers, insurance companies, and the general public.

The core of this book is the utilization of case studies to delineate health benefits and risks associated with medical intervention. We believe that the BRCT is generically applicable and its use could serve to further efforts toward the development of a universal decision aid. Since more emphasis is being placed on confronting escalating medical costs, acknowledged over-treatment and its iatrogenic consequences, the focus of this book is timely.

Effective use of decision aids requires an acknowledgment by physicians that the benefits from screening tests and other medical intervention remain controversial. Open and objective statements about such uncertainty are essential if we are to find a 'path forward'. Further, it is hoped that a clear and objective decision aid will encourage patients to fully participate in decision making and physicians to willingly discuss risks and benefits of tests and other procedures.

Since stories are essential to human experience, we shall be telling them in this book. The use of statistics will be minimal. Emphasis will be placed on graphics, since we believe a picture is worth more than 10,000 words—in our view, the graphic should do the math for patients. We stress the need to ask the 'right' questions. It has been our experience that if patients ask the 'right' questions, physicians will respond openly and honestly.

Notice: This book is not intended as a medical guide to self-treatment. The information of a medical nature in this book is meant to help you make informed decisions about your health by providing a more careful and complete understanding of benefits, risks, and uncertainty. If you suspect you need medical treatment, you should discuss it with your primary care physician. If you are being treated for a medical condition or are on medication, do not change your treatment program without discussing it with your doctor.

Baltimore, MD, USA   Erik Rifkin
                                                                                                          Andrew Lazris

Acknowledgments

We would like to thank colleagues and friends who were willing to share their insights with us regarding the interpretation of health benefits and risks and how doctors and patients can make the right medical choices together. Their views and perspectives improved this book and we are grateful for their encouragement.

We would also like to thank everyone who was willing to take the time and effort to provide candid and critical comments regarding the purpose, focus, format, and content of this book. We are particularly indebted to Elaine, Cathy, and Jill for reading through our drafts and making changes and suggestions which were invaluable and very much appreciated. We were fortunate to be able to call upon Kris Rifkin, a graphic designer, to professionally design and prepare the many Benefit/Risk Characterization Theaters.

Had it not been for vision and determination of professionals in the medical community advocating for patient-centered care and the use of absolute, rather than relative risks, this book would not have been possible. We are in their debt.

Finally, a special thanks to Dr. Tom Finucane for preparing a thoughtful and instructive Foreword to our book.

This book would not have been possible without the help of all the individuals named above.

About the Authors

Erik Rifkin is an environmental scientist who has had over 35 years of experience in characterizing human health and ecological risks from exposure to contaminants in soil, aquatic ecosystems, air and sediments. He has provided assistance and guidance to federal and state regulatory agencies, corporations, NGOs and the public in assessing risks associated with exposure to metals and organic pollutants in environmental media. In addition to publishing articles in peer-reviewed journals, Dr. Rifkin is a coauthor of the book, *The Illusion of Certainty-Health Benefits and Risks*, published by Springer in June 2007. His professional activities have underscored the importance of the communication of health risks and benefits to impacted groups.

Andrew Lazris is a practicing Internal Medicine physician with 25 years of experience. He is an honors history graduate from Brown University, having received his medical degree from Albert Einstein College of Medicine, and Board Certified in Internal Medicine after completing his residency at University of Virginia Hospital. He currently is the medical director of several geriatric long-term care facilities, gives regular talks in the community about health and medical issues, and directs Personal Physician Care in Columbia. He has published two fiction novels, and recently published *Curing Medicare* about the geriatric health care crisis. He is married with three kids and lives in Columbia, Maryland.

Contents

Part I   Setting the Stage

1   Shared Decision Making 3
  References 8

2   Decision Aids 9
  References 11

3   Towards a Universal Decision Aid 13
  Benefits from Reducing Blood Serum Cholesterol 14
  Absolute vs Relative Risks 16
  Acceptable Individual Risks 19
  References 20

4   Involving the Patient in Decision Making 21
  The Abyss of Uncertainty 23
  Sensible Assessments Made Easy 24
  A Patient-Centered Approach 25

5   BRCTs 27

Part II   Case Studies: Health Benefits and Risks

6   Breast Cancer Screening: Mammograms 33
  A. Key Questions 34
  B. Risks and Benefits 34
  BRCTs: Breast Cancer Screening: Mammograms 35
  C. Discussion 39
  References 40

7   Colon Cancer Screening with Colonoscopy 43
      A. Key Questions 44
      B. Risks and Benefits 44
      BRCTs: Colon Cancer Screening with Colonoscopy 45
      C. Discussion 48
      References 49

8   Prostate Cancer Screening 51
      A. Key Questions 52
      B. Risks and Benefits of Prostate Screening 52
      BRCTs: Prostate Cancer Screening 54
      C. Discussion 58
      References 61

9   Screening for Lung Cancer with Spiral CT 63
      A. Key Questions 64
      B. Risks and Benefits 64
      BRCTs: Screening for Lung Cancer with Spiral CT 66
      C. Discussion 69
      References 72

10   Health Effects of Smoking 73
      A. Key Questions 74
      B. Risks and Benefits 74
      BRCTs: Health Effects of Smoking 76
      C. Discussion 80
      References 82

11   Exercise Stress Tests 83
      A. Key Questions 84
      B. Risks and Benefits 84
      BRCTs: Exercise Stress Tests 86
      C. Discussion 90
      References 93

12   The Use of Warfarin in Atrial Fibrillation 95
      A. Key Questions 96
      B. Risks and Benefits 97
      BRCTs: The Use of Warfarin in Atrial Fibrillation 98
      C. Discussion 101
      References 103

13   Aspirin for Prevention of Heart Disease and Stroke 105
      A. Key Questions 106
      B. Risks and Benefits 106
      BRCTs: Aspirin for Prevention of Heart Disease and Stroke 108
      C. Discussion 111
      References 113

14   Screening for Carotid Disease in Asymptomatic Patients 115
      A. Key Questions 116
      B. Risks and Benefits 116
      BRCTs: Screening for Carotid Disease in Asymptomatic Patients 117
      C. Discussion 121
      References 122

15   Cholesterol Screening 125
      A. Key Questions 126
      B. Benefits and Risks 126
      BRCT: Cholesterol Screening 128
      C. Discussion 130
      References 132

16   Statins, Cholesterol, and Coronary Heart Disease 133
      A. Key Questions 134
      B. Risks and Benefits 134
      BRCTS: Statins, Cholesterol, and Coronary Heart Disease 136
      C. Discussion 141
      Primary Prevention Studies 143
      Secondary Prevention Studies 143
      References 144

17   Annual Exam 147
      A. Key Questions 148
      B. Risks and Benefits 148
      BRCTs: Annual Exam 150
      C. Discussion 154
      References 159

18   Screening for and Treating Dementia 161
      A. Key Questions 162
      B. Risks and Benefits 162
      BRCTs: Screening for and Treating Dementia 164
      C. Discussion 168
      References 170

19   Osteoporosis: Bone Density Testing and Drug Treatment 173
      A. Key Questions 174
      B. Risks and Benefits 174
      BRCTs: Osteoporosis: Bone Density Testing and Drug Treatment 176
      C. Discussion 179
      References 182

20 Osteoporosis: Calcium and Vitamin D 183
   A. Key Questions 184
   B. Risks and Benefits 184
   BRCTs: Osteoporosis: Calcium and Vitamin D 185
   C. Discussion 189
   References 191

21 Estrogen Replacement Therapy 193
   A. Key Questions 194
   B. Risks and Benefits 194
   BRCTs: Estrogen Replacement Therapy 196
   C. Discussion 199
   References 201

22 Vitamins and Supplements 203
   A. Key Questions 204
   B. Risks and Benefits 204
   BRCTs: Vitamins and Supplements... 205
   C. Discussion 208
   References 211

23 MRI and Back Pain 213
   A. Key Questions 214
   B. Risks and Benefits 214
   BRCTs: MRI and Back Pain... 215
   C. Discussion 218
   References 219

24 Antibiotics in Sinusitis and Bronchitis 221
   A. Key Questions 222
   B. Risks and Benefits 222
   BRCTs: Antibiotics in Sinusitis and Bronchitis 223
   C. Discussion 227
   References 228

25 Final Thoughts 229

Erratum to E1

Index 233

Part I
Setting the Stage

Chapter 1
Shared Decision Making

As soon as I heard his voice, I knew something was wrong. Usually, when my dad called, he was self-confident and wanted to assertively explain why the US policy toward some foreign country was misguided and would have draconian ramifications if implemented or why labor unions needed to reassert themselves. But this time his voice was subdued and shaky and the purpose of his call was to ask me for a favor.

My father had his annual physical and his doctor informed him that his prostate specific antigen (PSA) levels were unacceptably high. He was told that he needed to schedule an appointment for a biopsy of his prostate gland ASAP to determine if he had prostate cancer. In response to what that would entail, my dad was told by his physician that the biopsy could be painful and could lead to some serious complications (e.g., recently it has been demonstrated that this procedure can result in an increased incidence of potentially lethal, difficult-to-treat bloodstream infections; so serious that urologists are reassessing when, how, and even if they should do the procedure). In response to dad's queries regarding whether this biopsy was absolutely necessary, his physician's unequivocal response was yes.

My father was anxious and upset and wanted to know if I would call his doctor to see if there were any reasonable alternatives. If he were younger and more robust, my dad would have looked into the possibility of options himself. By nature he was a contrarian and never really obsessed health issues. But things had changed.

The year was 1993, my father was 81 years old and he had been diagnosed as having terminal emphysema. There was little doubt that his condition was due to smoking three packs of unfiltered cigarettes for over 70 years. He was on oxygen and told that he had, at most, 2 years to live. He was understandably beaten down and in need of some support and assistance.

I told him that I believed he should forgo the biopsy. I didn't go into any detail but voiced, as tactfully as I could, that his current condition precluded any need to get a biopsy of his prostate. Further, I informed my dad that elevated PSA levels were not a surrogate for prostate cancer. He told me he respected my views regarding this mat-

© Springer International Publishing Switzerland 2015
E. Rifkin, A. Lazris, *Interpreting Health Benefits and Risks*,
DOI 10.1007/978-3-319-11544-3_1

ter but needed to have his doctor state that it was alright to skip the biopsy. I said I understood (particularly since I was not a physician) and would make the call.

Later that day I was about to pick up the phone but decided to first reflect on how I should approach my dad's doctor. I had previously met him and thought that he was bright and answered questions honestly and directly. That being said, it was also clear to me that my father's physician was hearing his patient's concerns and preferences but not listening. This doctor was relying on protocol—if PSA is elevated, the next step is to recommend a biopsy. This is the next step, regardless of a patient's unique circumstances or concerns.

The distinction between hearing and listening is a critical one and needs to be understood if we are to achieve the goals of empowering patients, shared decision making (SDM), patient-centered care and effective communication with patients. Hearing is simply the act of perceiving sound by the ear. The ability to hear is critical to understanding the world around us and picking up sound and attaching meaning to it is a complex process. If you are not hearing-impaired, hearing simply happens. Listening, however, is something you consciously choose to do. Listening requires concentration so that your brain processes meaning from words and sentences—listening leads to learning.

Most people tend to be "hard of listening" rather than "hard of hearing." If you are "hard of listening," SDM is not difficult, it is virtually impossible. When I was growing up, my entire family was "hard of listening." Each of us perceived our views to be closer to God and could not wait to interrupt, jump in, and pontificate on why our answers were the right ones. There was not much listening going on but the consequences were not very serious.

On the other hand, if a patient is anxious and justifiably disturbed about a suggestion for a specific form of medical intervention and a physician has a preconceived idea regarding what constitutes "the right answers," grave consequences may result. The primary difference between the sense of hearing and the skill of listening is attention.

How difficult it is to listen when one's thoughts are elsewhere. Such as: what are the ramifications if protocols are not followed to the letter; I'm running 45 min late for my next appointment, and don't have time for a debate with my patient; if I had a high PSA, I would get the biopsy. A recent report published by the Institute of Medicine [1] confirms the critical importance of active listening, "The doctor also needs to listen to you so he or she understands your values, preferences, and goals. This is important because every patient is different, and when there are options, it is important for the doctor to know what is important to you"

Fortunately, we can train ourselves to listen by paying attention, a generically important concept which also happens to be directly applicable to the relatively new paradigm of patient-centered care. It certainly was relevant to my father's situation. The call I made to my dad's doctor was returned two days later. I thanked this physician for his time and told him that my father had asked me to call regarding his recommendation to have a biopsy based on elevated levels of PSA. Initially, his tone clearly indicated that he had little interest in discussing this decision with me. Undaunted, I told him that the call would only take a few minutes and that I would not have contacted him but my father was deeply disturbed about this biopsy and potential ramifications.

I asked him if he would take a minute or two to assess the likelihood that concerns associated with prostate cancer were meaningful, given my father's condition. This physician knew that my dad's health was deteriorating rapidly and the prognosis of 2 years was now overly optimistic. In light of that situation, I asked him to explain the rationale for his decision to suggest a biopsy to assess my dad's prostate gland. Finally, I informed him that my strong recommendation was that my father not be subjected to this biopsy or any other medical intervention associated with prostate cancer.

Upon further reflection, my dad's doctor said he did not disagree with my logic and asked if there were anything else to talk about since he was very busy. "Just one more thing" I replied, "please call my father and let him know you have changed your mind"—after a pause, he said OK. My dad was grateful and was now able to focus on issues relevant to the time he had left on this earth.

Of course, I was pleased with the outcome. But I did not say what was really on my mind, because if I had, the result may have been different. Given his condition, I would like to have asked this doctor why it was necessary to determine levels of PSA in my father's blood in the first place. Why did not a conversation occur about the course of treatment before the needle punctured my dad's arm? Why didn't the doctor attempt to address what was obviously a high level of uncertainty and apprehension? And, why wasn't my dad given information empowering him to share, in a meaningful way, in any decision regarding medical intervention? Why wasn't there any SDM?

This situation reminded me of my favorite "Far Side" cartoon which shows a man admonishing his dog—"Okay, Ginger! I've had it! You stay out of the garbage!" But Ginger only hears, "Blah blah Ginger blah blah blah blah Ginger..." Patients' hear physicians and nurses in a similar fashion, "Blah blah blah cholesterol blah blah heart attack blah blah stroke." (Same analogy was used recently in the Opinion Pages of the NYT) [2]. SDM has been defined as a collaborative process that encourages a patient and his physician to jointly participate in making health care decisions. As noted above, effective SDM will require open communication and listening.

Another prerequisite for successful SDM is that patients understand health risks and benefits associated with any medical intervention. Further, patients want clear, concise, and understandable information regarding the effectiveness of a procedure or treatment and its applicability to their personal condition and social situation [3]. SDM also requires doctors to take into consideration what constitutes each patient's level of acceptable risks.

One common scenario where this plays out is in the area of screening tests. Physicians use clinical guidelines or protocols to determine when screening tests such as mammograms, pap smears, cholesterol levels, PSA blood tests, bone density tests, colonoscopies, and other lab tests should be performed. These guidelines are often dictated by insurance, such as Medicare, or are outlined by such groups as the American Cancer Society and the US Preventive Services Task Force.

While the guidelines mandate or recommend certain screening tests, rarely do they present information in a way that helps doctors explain the risks and benefits of those procedures to a particular patient.

For a variety of reasons, both doctors and patients are currently limited in their ability to determine the appropriateness and frequency of screening tests. Patients have access to the same recommendations, but far more often they are influenced by the media, common lore, and by insurance reimbursements. Decisions are rarely based on a clear understanding of what constitutes acceptable risks and benefits of a certain test; rather the physician dictates which tests are necessary, or the patients request the tests he/she believes to be necessary.

Often patients come in for their annual exam expecting me to order the requisite screening tests. When I do discuss each test with them, rather than relying on what a clinical guideline declares, my patients gain more insight into whether they really want to pursue the screening test. I have had multiple patients who dread getting a colonoscopy but who believe that they must do so, something that had been reinforced by other doctors without any discussion about the risks and benefits, and by their own preconceived notions.

When I do share with them how often a colonoscopy may prevent cancer in people without symptoms, and how often the same test can cause harm, some of my patients elect to defer the test, while others still believe it to be necessary. With either decision, the patient and doctor both used real data, rather than a perception of what must be done, to reach a more satisfying conclusion.

The concept that doctors and patients should make medical choices together is relatively new. While it's hard to pinpoint the beginning of movements, the Karen Ann Quinlan case in 1968 forced the medical community to realize that the decision making process would become more cumbersome in the future.

This highly publicized case regarding who has the right to decide if and when this young woman in a coma should die, involved her family, politicians, the medical community, attorneys, philosophers, and the general public. It galvanized groups with strong convictions regarding patient involvement in making medical choices; e.g., to share their views and perspectives with the general public.

Forty three years later there has been a dramatic increase in the level of interest and involvement by private and public institutions in programs and projects associated with patient-centered care. This is due, in part, to the passage of the Affordable Care Act (ACA). There is considerably more awareness today of the need for doctor/patient collaboration than there was just a few years ago.

As noted in the preface, ACA* has a number of provisions which are designed to address concerns caregivers and patients face when making critical health care choices without key information that would help them make better decisions.

---

*Unfortunately, these goals and objectives appear to be antithetical to other provisions of the ACA which will disrupt the concept of individualized care. The ACA relies on clinical practice guidelines which set very concrete protocols regarding treatment and testing. Adherence to these practice guidelines are barriers to SDM and will significantly limit the ability of physicians to practice individualized care.

So, in light of all this good news, are doctors and patients listening and communicating with one another? While patient-centered care has become a high profile issue, the answer is not yet. As is the case with other complex and controversial issues, well-intentioned initiatives, momentum, and positive rhetoric are necessary, but not sufficient, to achieve success. Major roadblocks remain before meaningful SDM can occur. According to Peter A. Ubel, MD (in his recently published book—*Critical Decisions—How You and Your Doctor Can Make the Right Medical Choices Together*) [4], "If we truly want to improve physician communication and bring new doctors into the profession who are ready and willing to work with activated patients, we need to pay attention not only to *who* we educate as physicians but also *how* we educate them."

In addition, recommendations regarding treatment for chronic health endpoints are, more often than not, replete with uncertainty and controversial. Definitions of basic terms (e.g., patient-centered care, empowering patients, evidence-based medicine, and comparative-effectiveness research) appear to reflect, to a large degree, the vested interest of those proffering the definition. Further, there is no agreed upon standard methodological approach for communicating health risk and benefit information to patients. Unless a consistent, logical, "universal" paradigm is defined and accepted, progress will be limited and inertia will become the norm.

There are also concerns regarding preconceived views and perspectives of patients. Many Americans generally believe that others should be responsible for their care. This mindset is antithetical to SDM and patient empowerment and, therefore, must be modified if patients want to have meaningful input in decisions regarding medical intervention. Not all patients want tests or drugs, but many do. So, physicians may well be responding to patient preference when making recommendations regarding tests and screening.

The growing groups of patients who want to be involved are left to sift through contradictory information to find the most "meaningful" health benefit and risk statistics presented to them by experts. The "worried well" can feel confused about what to do regarding medical recommendations. Individuals who are not obviously ill or in danger, but aging, reading articles about medical interventions in newspapers and magazines, perhaps with a few aches and pains, maybe lost a friend or two through cancer or a heart attack, are uncertain about what, if anything, they should be doing.

A recent example of this occurred when most major newspapers published the results of a study suggesting that screening smokers and ex-smokers for lung cancer with annual spiral CT scans reduces the rate of lung cancer death by approximately 25 %. Several of my patients who formerly smoked, and who feared cancer, came to me requesting a CT scan. At the time, most insurance still did not pay for the scan, and groups such as the US Preventive Services Task Force had only recently recommended lung cancer screening, but the visits afforded me an opportunity to discuss the screening test with them.

Several important numbers were not mentioned in the plethora of news coverage that convinced my patients that they needed this test. Out of 1,000 people receiving CT scans every year, how many deaths were averted? How often did the tests show an abnormal finding that, after other testing, was found to be non-cancerous? What was the risk of getting the CT, including the risk of unnecessary harmful procedures and treatments for what proved not to be cancer? Having a discussion using real information like this helps to put sensationalism in health care to rest; doctors and patients can sift through meaningful numbers to reach a decision that makes sense for that particular patient. Of course, it is often easier just to order the test and not discuss its ramifications. *In the end, though, the time spent talking about a particular test or intervention can save time down the road, and can lead to a much more satisfying interaction.*

Doctors and patients are faced with a daunting task: Find the best way to make the right medical choices together. Any feasible method must surmount real constraints on physicians and patients alike. Many factors contribute to our being over-tested and over-medicated. American doctors might be more in the habit of prescribing medications instead of counseling patients on behaviors that might reduce the need for medication in the first place. What is missing from the discussion is how some patients are anxious, deeply anxious, about their overall health.

Nevertheless, it's not unreasonable to assume that more and more physicians are embracing the concept of SDM and they are committed to allotting the time necessary to empower patients to become participants in the decision making process. But embracing a concept does not automatically result in successful implementation. The seminal question remains: *How do physicians and patients reach common ground!* One of the ways to achieve that objective is by using decision aids.

References

1. Alston, C., Paget, L., Halvorson, G., Novelli, B., Guest, J., McCabe, P., Hoffman, K., Koepke, C., Simon, M., Sutton, S., Okun, S., Wicks, P., Undem, T., Rohrbach, V., Von Kohorn, I. (2012). *Communicating with patients on health care evidence*. Discussion Paper, Institute of Medicine, Washington, DC.
2. Brown, T. (2014). *Lost in clinical translation*. NYT Opinion Pages, February 8, 2014.
3. Huckman, R. S., & Kelley, M. A. (2013). Public reporting, consumerism, and patient empowerment. *The New England Journal of Medicine, 369*, 1875–1877.
4. Ubel, P. A. (2012). *Critical decisions: how you and your doctor can make the right medical choices together*. New York: HarperOne. 360 pp.

Chapter 2
Decision Aids

Decision aids are tools designed to enable effective shared decision-making (SDM). They are used to assist patients in considering options associated with medical intervention. They describe where choice exists and where there is an option of taking no action. They are used to improve the communication process between doctor and patient.

These aids or tools assist patients in considering alternatives regarding short, intermediate, and long-term outcomes which have relevant consequences. They support the SDM process of constructing preferences and eventual decision-making, suitable to their individual situation [1]. While these interventions have been available in a variety of forms for over 25 years, there is evidence that the use of decision aids has not become routine practice for most physicians [2].

Many of the groups and institutions supporting the use of decision support interventions are based in North America, including *The Informed Medical Decisions Foundation* and *Healthwise*. There are also many active research groups in the field, including the *University of Ottawa, Dartmouth College, Cardiff University,* and *Hamburg* (A comprehensive collection of decision aids can be found at *www.Med-Decs.org*) [3].

There are many ways in which decision aids can, and have been, be used [1]. Evidence from randomized trials has been summarized in a Cochrane Collaboration systematic review [4]. This review confirmed that decision aids, when used, performed better than usual care interventions in terms of: (1) higher level of patient understanding; (2) higher level of SDM; and (3) reduced conflict related to feeling unclear about personal values. More specifically, exposure to decision aids demonstrated reduced rates of elective invasive surgery in favor of more conservative options.

There has been an increase in use of decision support, and a global interest in developing these interventions exists among both for-profit and not-for-profit organizations [5]. There is also evidence that the number of patients using decision aids has steadily increased over the years, both in Europe and the US.

© Springer International Publishing Switzerland 2015
E. Rifkin, A. Lazris, *Interpreting Health Benefits and Risks*,
DOI 10.1007/978-3-319-11544-3_2

While decision aids are not common, they are considered to be a key component of SDM. However, a majority of patients have no knowledge of them. As a result, most patients facing important medical decisions continue to assent to the suggestions of their doctor without using a decision aid [3].

While the reasons for this situation are manifold and difficult to quantify, the current quality of decision aids and medical community resistance to their use are probably key factors. The development of decision aids can be characterized as a dynamic process, which has not come close to meeting its potential. Decision aids will not achieve their maximal value if the only thing they accomplish is to increase patient knowledge; information does not necessarily lead to triggering SDM.

Many of my patients do come in with information that they obtained from newspapers, the internet, or other doctors. That information alone is not sufficient to help them make an informed decision. One common example of this relates to Alzheimer's disease, a horrible form of dementia that people will do anything to treat.

Many family members of demented patients have read everything they can about the disease. They have visited neurologists and other experts and have pursued every treatment available. There are medicines for dementia that can, according to many experts, help mitigate the disease's symptoms.

When side effects cause patients to stop a dementia drug, or if a patient refuses to take it, the spouse, knowing how important the drug is from all that he/she read and was told, feels devastated. But such drugs are much more nuanced in their impact, as we will discuss, and often other more mundane interventions can have more profound effects on the progression of dementia. Simply having facts and an arbitrary base of knowledge regarding the disease and its treatment does not help such patients and families reach informed decisions with their doctors.

In order to remedy this situation, it will be necessary to develop a universally accepted paradigm for decision aids with internationally accepted standards. This will result in the larger medical community being on "the same page" and will provide patients with a consistent and objective approach for all health endpoints.

As was noted above, there is general agreement that positive benefits result from the use of decision aids. That having been said, it is also acknowledged that these tools require upgrading if they are to be accepted by large numbers of physicians and patients [6, 7]. One of the reasons this has become a glacial process may be related to financial incentives to perform unnecessary procedures. There is another more subtle, but very significant, issue. Before patient empowerment can be achieved, doctors need to accept the notion that it is the patient who makes the final decision.

To facilitate this transition, emphasis would need to be placed on the concepts of patient-preference and a patient's definition of acceptable risk. There appear to be encouraging signs lately as patients appear to be positively predisposed to SDM. A recent discussion paper released by the Institute of Medicine [8] states, "... people recognize the common-sense value of sharing information to improve health and health-care – and possibly that there is a thirst in the general population for care improvement through data sharing. Physicians also need to be open to modifying behavior regarding the adherence to following standard procedures."

A common example of this is the practice of ordering routine cardiac testing. In my practice, many of my patients see cardiologists regularly. Some of these patients had heart attacks in the distant past, have ongoing stable heart disease, or have no heart disease but want to be proactive. Very often they are told that they need to get periodic screenings with stress tests, echocardiograms, or Holter monitors. These tests are not based on new or changed symptoms, but rather are done fairly routinely as screening tests. Most of my patients accede to the tests without question; they assume that if the doctor wants the test, there is good reason for it. Many also believe that getting the test will help them avoid a heart attack.

Recently one of my patients asked me why he needed to get the stress test. I told him that I was unsure, but I did tell him that in the majority of people who die suddenly from a heart attack a stress test would have been normal and not predicted risk. I also told him that many abnormal stress tests in asymptomatic people are false positives; they pick up problems that are not clinically significant and that will not lead to heart attacks if left alone, but which can lead to unnecessary invasive tests and treatments when discovered. When the patient subsequently talked to his cardiologist about his concerns, both agreed to defer the test.

At a minimum, patient decision aids should:

- Provide information about options and their associated relevant outcomes;
- Help patients to personalize this information and understand that they can be involved in decision-making;
- Assist patients in understanding the scientific uncertainties inherent in most choices;
- Clearly present potential benefits relative to potential harms;
- Help patients gain skills in the steps of collaborative decision-making.

A pivotal question is how to prepare patients for taking an active role in determining what form of medical intervention, if any, is best for each individual. Once decision aids are successful in preparing patients for this role, they will play an essential part in empowering patients. Key to achieving this goal is overall agreement on criteria which would constitute a meaningful decision aid. While few disagree with this need, controversy associated with the definition of the term SDM and the inherent inertia in large public institutions may continue to slow down this process.

References

1. Elwyn, G., Frosch, D., Volandes, A., Edwards, A., & Montori, V. (2009). *Investing in deliberation: Defining and developing decision support interventions for people facing difficult health decisions.* White Paper Series. Gaithersburg, Maryland, USA: John M Eisenberg Center for Clinical Decisions and Communication.
2. Gravel, K., Légaré, F., & Graham, I. D. (2006). Barriers and facilitators to implementing shared decision-making in clinical practice: A systematic review of health professionals' perceptions. *Implementation Science, 1,* 16. doi:10.1186/1748-5908-1-16. PMC 1586024. PMID 16899124.

3. Ubel, P. A. (2012). *Critical decisions: How you and your doctor can make the right medical choices together*. New York: HarperOne. 360 pp.

4. Stacey, D., Bennett, C. L., Barry, M. J. et al. (2011). Decision aids for people facing health treatment or screening decisions. *Cochrane Database of Systematic Reviews, 3,* CD001431. doi:10.1002/14651858.CD001431.pub3. PMID 19588325.

5. O'Connor, A. M., Wennberg, J. E., Legare, F. et al. (2007). Toward the 'tipping point': Decision aids and informed patient choice. *Health Aff (Millwood) 26*(3), 716–725. doi:10.1377/hlthaff.26.3.716. PMID 17485749.

6. Elwyn, G., O'Connor, A., Stacey, D. et al. (2006). Developing a quality criteria framework for patient decision aids: Online international Delphi consensus process. *British Medical Journal, 333*(7565), 417. doi:10.1136/bmj.38926.629329.AE. PMC 1553508. PMID 16908462.

7. Elwyn, G., O'Connor, A. M., Bennett, C. et al. (2009). Assessing the quality of decision support technologies using the International Patient Decision Aid Standards instrument (IPDASi). *PLoS One, 4*(3), e4705. doi:10.1371/journal.pone.0004705. PMC 2649534. PMID 19259269.

8. Alston, C., Paget, L., Halvorson, G., Novelli, B., Guest, J., McCabe, P., Hoffman, K., Koepke, C., Simon, M., Sutton, S., Okun, S., Wicks, P., Undem, T., Rohrbach, V., & Von Kohorn, I. (2012). *Communicating with patients on health care evidence*. Discussion Paper, Institute of Medicine, Washington, D.C. http://www.iom.edu/evidence.

Chapter 3
Towards a Universal Decision Aid

Prior to the turn of the century there were less than two dozen decision aids; now the number exceeds 500. Several decision aids can be found on the internet, however, many do not cite evidence sources, have presentations which are partial, and lack agreed upon quality criteria. In order to determine whether patient decision aids achieve their primary objective—to improve the quality of decisions—future decision aids need to be based on outcomes.

Decision aids may include various types of media, flyers, and brochures. The assortment of aids currently being used has resulted in the absence of a uniform set of criteria or standards which are needed to ensure the effectiveness and increased use of future decision aids. Our experience suggests that if these aids were improved they would be viewed more positively and, therefore, more likely to be used by physicians and patients alike.

Patients need to be comfortable with the format of a decision aid. Information needs to be presented in terms and in a setting that is familiar to patients—the presentation needs to "feel" right. This format should show patients, as simply and effortlessly as possible, what an act, procedure, or drug means in terms of their own health objectives and their quality of life. The standard approach of flashing traditional pie charts or line graphs, which demand considerable statistical sophistication to fully understand, is not going to resonate with most patients—or physicians for that matter.

Decision aids should be designed to generate a conversation between doctor and patient. In spite of the controversy and absence of certainty associated with medical intervention, these aids should enable physicians and patients to take the first step towards reaching "common ground." Since most patients are not physicians or scientists, equations, calculations, percentages, or technical text would add to their confusion.

Since a picture is worth 1,000 words (at least), what is also needed is a simple, straight-forward graphic which presents, on one page, a clear and objective picture of health benefits and risks associated with different kinds of medical intervention.

© Springer International Publishing Switzerland 2015
E. Rifkin, A. Lazris, *Interpreting Health Benefits and Risks*,
DOI 10.1007/978-3-319-11544-3_3

This decision aid should be generically applicable and able to address a variety of types and forms of suggested procedures.

A visual aid depicting recognizable or accustomed situations could be very effective in achieving this purpose. Information could be framed in a manner that enables people to relate health statistics and risk analyses to accustomed experiences. It would critical that information contained in any decision aid not be biased in the direction of risk aversion or risk acceptance.

In order for this communication tool to be successful, it should include a visual display that enables the reader to look at an image and be able to readily determine risks and benefits from screening tests (e.g., colonoscopy, PSA test, mammogram, cholesterol), drugs (e.g., statins, Warfarin), and procedures for a number of health endpoints. The selected image should be able to demonstrate at a glance that a 1 in 10 risk is very different from a 1 in 1,000 risk.

We would like to suggest a unique graphic providing standardization which both lay people and the medical community could share when discussing courses of action. Given that we are in an era when patients are compulsively surfing the internet—it would also make sense for all medical articles to include a uniform graphic to express the meaning of their findings to a lay audience and the media.

Most of us are familiar with the crowd in a typical theater as a graphic illustration of a population grouping. It occurred to us that a theater seating chart could be used to objectively characterize and communicate health benefits and risks. We call our decision aid a *Benefit/Risk Characterization Theater (BRCT)*. We have successfully used it to assist patients in determining: their level of acceptable risk; if the benefits of intervention outweigh the risks; who should make the final decision regarding medical intervention; and, whether the decision is evidence-based. With a seating capacity of 1,000, our BRCT can make shared decision making a straight forward and positive experience for doctor and patient.

Below is an example of a BRCT (Fig. 3.1) which illustrates the benefits of cholesterol screening. Emphasis is placed on death from coronary heart disease (CHD) as the end point, not cholesterol levels. Patients can readily see themselves in this BRCT and, based on their level of acceptable risk, decide whether a 1 in 1,000 death benefit from screening constitutes the need for medical intervention (e.g., statins, restrictive diet).

This format requires the use of absolute values and eliminates the use of relative risks (see below), which often results in the dissemination of misinformation. Presenting this information on one page affords physicians the opportunity to quickly summarize essential information and effectively communicate with their patients.

Benefits from Reducing Blood Serum Cholesterol

The BRCT graphic virtues are instantly obvious. Traditional statistical charts rarely convey the often random pattern in which diseases or conditions manifest themselves. Seating patterns show that an illness, for instance, may strike one person,

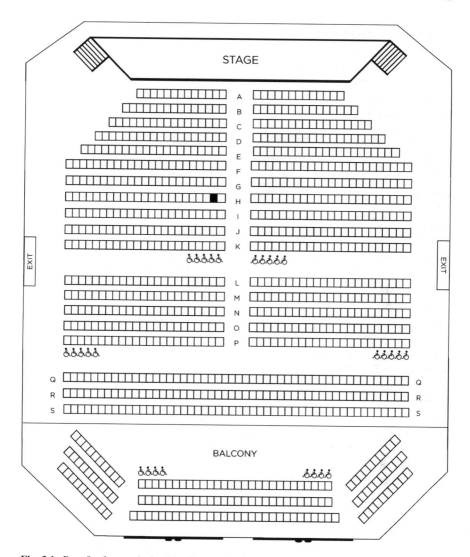

Fig. 3.1 Benefits from reducing blood serum cholesterol. If there were 1,000 people sitting in a theater with significantly elevated cholesterol levels of 280 mg, there would be one additional death, represented by one darkened seat, per year from coronary heart disease as compared to 1,000 people with normal cholesterol

and not his/her neighbor, who has the same habits, age, and/or sex. The inclusion of BRCTs in peer reviewed articles would enable physicians, patients, and the media to objectively assess risks and benefits from medical intervention. Perhaps this approach would encourage pharmaceutical companies and the press to use absolute values and not relative risks when reporting on findings associated with health risks and benefits.

Absolute vs Relative Risks

There are a number of criteria a decision aid must meet to improve the SDM process. A key, if not the key, criterion is to insure that health risks and benefits are presented to patients as absolute risks (as is the case in our BRCTs) and *never as relative risks.*

This is a critically important issue and a brief presentation here is warranted. Absolute risks and benefits reflect *the number of people who will get a disease, compared to the total number of people being considered.* Absolute benefits and risks are the difference between two groups.

In Fig. 3.1, the BRCT demonstrates that 1 additional individual (represented by one darkened seat) in 1,000 with elevated cholesterol will die from CHD when compared with 1,000 individuals with normal cholesterol (see Chapter 15 on Cholesterol Screening). These are *absolute* values and, therefore, compare the number of people who will get a disease with the *total* number of people being considered. Such a graphic enables patients to have a solid and tangible starting point, to discuss acceptable risks and benefits in the context of their own value systems.

While one patient may perceive the single blackened seat sufficient to warrant the use of cholesterol lowering drugs, another patient may dismiss the intervention as trivial. In both cases, the patient receives identical and easily digestible information from a physician and then makes an informed decision.

A good example of this pertains to the annual exam. Often my patients come to me once a year expecting a complete physical. The definition of such an exam varies from patient to patient; some want me to examine every part of them, others expect blood tests and EKGs, still others seek a wide array of testing and screening in addition to the exam. Recent data has questioned the value of an annual exam, but patients still appreciate it and doctors typically perform it.

One elderly patient came in to tell me that she was not satisfied by my recent annual exam; her prior doctor had been much more thorough. I asked her what she wanted me to do, and she told me: I had not ordered a urine test or EKG, listened to her carotid arteries, fully examined her skin, sent her for a bone density scan, or done a rectal exam. Having been researching for this book, I happened to have BRCTs for each of these tests, and I shared them with my patient, including both the absolute benefits and risks of what she requested.

The discussion took no more than ten minutes, and in the end she agreed with my decision to eschew certain parts of the exam, although she wished I had discussed it with her at the time. In fact, she was absolutely correct: I had used data to make the decision *for* her and not *with* her, which only led her to be upset. By sharing the BRCTs she was able now to make her own decision, and if that decision verged from my own, then I knew at least she was basing it on real and pertinent information. Luckily, though, we both were in agreement.

Unfortunately, researchers, doctors, newspapers, radio, TV, web designers and pharmaceutical companies frequently (almost always) frame their messages using relative risks. This results in the public receiving misinformation that dramatically exaggerates and distorts health risks and benefits associated with medical intervention. So, what are relative risks and why are using them in communicating health benefits and risks an anathema?

Relative risks[*] are almost always presented as percentages. For example, a pharmaceutical company announces that a cancer drug reduces death from liver cancer by **50 %**. Or, a prominent newspaper reports that not having a colonoscopy will increase the risk of getting colon cancer by **20–25 %**. Or, the chief scientist of a breast imaging company states that annual mammograms reduce rates of breast cancer by **30–35 %** and four major newspapers pick up the story and include these percentages in the story headline.

What do those percentages mean? Are those results meaningful? *While these percentages appear to be significant, the bottom line is there is insufficient information to make an informed decision.* And generally speaking when you see percentages when discussing health risks and benefits they are, to all intents and purposes, meaningless and hollow. But how can that be the case? Perhaps a few examples will help.

Let's say, in a hypothetical example, that a reporter for a prominent newspaper compared annual deaths from drowning in two groups of 100,000 men and women. The first group of 100,000 was composed of recreational swimmers and the second group was made up of swimmers who were also SCUBA divers. The story headline read, *SCUBA Diving Increases Death Rate by 50 %.* What does that mean? It certainly sounds like SCUBA divers are at great risk and should think about doing something else. But as it turns out two individuals out of 100,000 SCUBA divers drowned and 1 out of 100,000 in the swimming group drowned annually. Relative risks, by definition, compare the 2 deaths to 1 death and come up with a 50 % increase.

But the absolute difference is 1/100,000 or 0.0001 %, i.e., 2 minus 1 in 100,000. It is unlikely that any SCUBA diver would be dissuaded by that small a risk. Therefore, without defining an established population (in this case 100,000) as a reference, percentages used to characterize risks are misleading and virtually useless.

In a second hypothetical example a researcher from an Ivy League school was interested in assessing the increased risk from exposure to lightening in Florida. He did some research and found that three individuals living in Florida out of a million were killed by lightening over a 5-year period. He compared those risks with individuals living in the Mid-Atlantic States where 2 individuals per million were killed by lightening over a 5-year period. This researcher chose to use relative risks to characterize the risks. So, his results were on the cover of a number of newspapers and on TV and the conclusion was: *There is a 33 % greater risk of being killed by lightening in Florida than in the Mid-Atlantic States*—(Comparison between 3 deaths and 2 deaths). Actually, there was 1 additional death in Florida for every

---

[*] *While Relative Risk Reduction is a useful yardstick for epidemiologists and public health officials, it should **never** be used by the public and physicians to assess the risks and benefits of medical intervention.*

1,000,000 people; an absolute risk of 1 in 1,000,000. That is hardly a reason to avoid moving to Florida.

It is a bit concerning that headlines which use relative risks probably sell more newspapers and get a higher TV rating. Pharmaceutical companies using relative risks to describe drug benefits and absolute risks to describe complications from drugs may realize greater profits.

Using the cholesterol BRCT example above, research has shown that 1,000 people with elevated cholesterol levels would have two deaths annually from CHD and 1,000 people with normal cholesterol would have 1 death annually from CHD. To calculate relative risks in this situation, focus would be on the 2 deaths compared to 1 death. The size of the group being studied would be ignored. Since 2 deaths is 50 % more than 1 death a pharmaceutical company could state the following; *Studies clearly demonstrate that lowering cholesterol reduced deaths from CHD by 50 %.* Sounds like a genuine medical breakthrough! It would seem that no matter what cholesterol lowering drugs cost and what side effects they may cause, you need to take them.

The point is that without an appropriate context, 50 % is a meaningless value for patients (in point of fact, a meaningless value for anyone). The result is that patients are bombarded with information that leads to exaggerated expectations of the benefits of medical intervention and the risks of not taking drugs.

The bottom line is that decision aids should never include information on relative risks in text, discussion, or illustrations. The inappropriateness of using relative risks to characterize health risks and benefits has been confirmed by prominent physicians. When discussing the use of relative risks, Dr. Gilbert Welch, Professor of Medicine, Dartmouth Institute for Health Policy and Clinical Practice states, "Relative change can dramatically exaggerate the underlying effect. It's a great way to scare people." He goes on to say, "Relative change also exaggerate effects in the other direction. It's a great way to make people believe there has been a medical breakthrough" [1].

Dr. Nortin Hadler, Professor of Medicine and Microbiology, University North Carolina, in his book *Worried Sick* states in capital letters; "NEVER LET ANYONE TALK OF RELATIVE RISK REDUCTION WITHOUT DEMANDING A STATEMENT OF ABSOLUTE-RISK REDUCTION." He also references a review of 359 studies of new treatments published in major medical journals which found that "the majority expressed and emphasized their results as 'relative risk' reduction." Dr. Hadler also emphasized the point that abstracts of peer reviewed articles, the section most likely to be read, generally contained misleading statistics—such as relative risks. In spite of the admonitions of Dr. Hadler and others, very little has changed over the past 6 years, since his book was published [2].

We agree with these medical professionals and others advocating for the use of absolute values when characterizing health risks and benefits. Unfortunately, in today's world, the vast majority of health information is disseminated by using relative risk numbers.

Acceptable Individual Risks

Organizations concerned with public health issues in the US (and other countries) want to reduce overall deaths nationwide (e.g., Centers for Disease Control, American Cancer Society, National Institutes of Health). As public health stewards, these groups report countrywide statistics on cancer, heart attacks, and other chronic conditions. Nationwide, deaths from heart attacks and colon, prostate, breast, and lung cancer exceed one million every year in the US alone. Gathering and interpreting this information is vital to the overall health of populations. *However, nationwide numbers are not particularly useful for individuals who are trying to understand their individual level of risk and/or benefits and decide if it's acceptable to them.*

If 50,000 people benefit from a certain intervention nationwide, that seems impressive. But if 2 out of every 1,000 people given that intervention benefit, while 50 out of every 1,000 can react poorly to the intervention, that information is far more meaningful to the individual patient having to make a decision.

We need a more accessible framework that enables us to comprehend health benefits in a more relevant, direct, and practical context. Overall health benefits to thousands of individuals in a population of hundreds of millions are hard to imagine. They translate poorly, if at all, at the personal level. We need to be able to obtain and interpret data which will permit us to make a decision based on our own individual level of acceptable risks.

Physicians and patients participating in the SDM process will need to acknowledge and address the *concept of individual acceptable risks*. Most definitions of SDM inherently assume that patient preferences, based on values, principles, tenets, bias, and so on, should play a major role in any final decision(s) on medical intervention. But, in order for patients and doctors to have a meaningful discussion of acceptable risk, they both need to openly recognize and accept this premise. Today in the US, the medical community has not successfully incorporated the concept of individual acceptable risk into the SDM process. In our view, use of BRCTs can assist in reaching that goal.

Encouraging patients to be screened for breast, colon, prostate, and other cancers presupposes that worthwhile national benefits will be derived from these screening programs. It has been determined that national benefits associated with cancer screening are substantial in certain instances. This determination is based on the values and perspectives of the organizations that manage these health issues. However, individual benefits, from the same screening tests, may be viewed as inconsequential by many patients (see Case Studies for screening tests below).

We have evidence that the BRCT is effective at removing obstacles that doctors and patients face when attempting to communicate about health risks and benefits associated with medical intervention. The utilization of a decision aid like the BRCT would, by definition, result in eliminating the use of relative values to explain health risks and benefits to patients. The goal would be to use a universal decision aid which could become standard practice in physician/patient interactions, and used routinely by medical journals, pharmaceutical companies, and the media.

References

1. Welch, H. G. (2012). *The problem is relative*. Huffington: Post blog.
2. Hadler, N. M. (2008). *Worried sick: A prescription for health in an overtreated America*. The Chapel Hill: University of North Carolina Press. 376 pp.

Chapter 4
Involving the Patient in Decision Making

As a physician who practices medicine daily, I am frequently faced with choices regarding appropriate medical care. I practice Internal Medicine, and the bulk of my patients are elderly. They have multiple chronic illnesses and are often on many medicines and supplements. Are all of those medicines necessary? How frequently should they be screened for cancer, tested for heart disease, or receive blood work? Which interventions are beneficial to their health, and just how beneficial are they? If beneficial, are there any untoward effects?

In an ideal world, physicians and patients would sit down and discuss these questions. We would run through the medicine lists, talk about screening, and review tests that may be appropriate. We would also discuss lifestyle changes that are beneficial. Of course, all of that takes time, and very often physicians are time constrained by economic and logistical reality. Also, the answers to most questions are nebulous and thus not amenable to a facile discussion. Rarely are there absolutes in health care delivery. Quite often it is far easier for the doctor to simply tell the patient what to do and avoid what can be an arduous conversation. Part of the difficulty arises from the fact that physicians and patients both have unique lenses that peer into the subtleties of medical issues, and neither has good tools to help drive a mutually beneficial discussion.

In the new world of medicine, spearheaded by the Affordable Care Act and Medicare reform, physicians are encouraged to follow clinical guidelines that suggest certain screening tests, procedures, and treatments, such as giving statin cholesterol medicines to people with diabetes, or ordering bone density tests on women over 65. As we shall see, the benefits of these and other tests and treatments are not as clear cut as the guidelines may suggest, and often after a rational discussion many of my patients chose to not pursue the intervention. Therefore, it is important that doctors and patients have tools with which to discuss these important issues, rather than to simply follow guidelines that may not be in concert with a patient's wishes.

© Springer International Publishing Switzerland 2015
E. Rifkin, A. Lazris, *Interpreting Health Benefits and Risks*,
DOI 10.1007/978-3-319-11544-3_4

Many of my patients derive medical information from both the lay press and the internet. The latter source is notoriously unreliable. Internet sources are not consistently screened for accuracy, and they often make very bold and simplistic proclamations that are so vague and erroneous that they obfuscate the truth. The lay press can be equally misleading. Often stories are simplified, and almost always their results are delivered in percentages of improvement/danger that represent relative risk.

As discussed, even very miniscule alterations in absolute risk from medical interventions can be magnified by relative risk calculations. Patients can be led to believe that certain tests or treatments are very effective, even if the efficacy is very small. Physicians also are fed information in a misleading format which can equally obscure complicated issues, since most medical studies present their conclusions through the window of relative risk.

Also impacting any doctor–patient discussion is the definition of screening tests. We will be discussing many screening tests in this book; tests performed on people without symptoms in an attempt to discover problems before they become serious. Such tests could include mammograms, colonoscopies, annual physical exams, exercise stress tests, and carotid ultrasounds. These are to be distinguished from disease-specific testing, such as ordering a stress test for a patient experiencing chest pain.

One peril of screening tests is that often they reveal a large number of false positive results. A test can be abnormal even in people without disease because the test itself is not very accurate. For instance, of all exercise stress tests that are positive, only a small number of those will be indicative of clinically relevant heart disease. A person with a positive stress test may have to undergo further testing, such as with catheterization, to ascertain whether he or she actually has heart disease, and may even have interventions with such modalities as stents and bypass surgery to "fix" problems that, if left alone, would have caused them no harm. These unnecessary procedures could potentially be dangerous, meaning that the screening test itself, due to its false positive finding, actually hurts the patient who received it. Also, such a person will now be labeled as having cardiac disease and treated with medicines unnecessarily, also potentially causing harm and even stress. In assessing the value of a screening test, then, the absolute rate of false positives, as well as their implications, should be discussed.

A similar difficulty with screening tests is the rate of false negatives. Screening tests are limited in their ability to detect the diseases for which they are searching. A test could be normal, but the patient may not be. For instance, a sizable number of people who die from heart disease have had normal exercise stress tests before their events. Therefore, the normal screening test gave them false assurance that they were disease free. Tests with a high absolute false negative number could also be problematic, and that information needs to be discussed.

When I first read *The Illusion of Certainty* (published by Springer in 2007) several years ago, and then met with the author Erik Rifkin, I was able to develop new tools with which to discuss complicated issues with my patients. The Risk Characterization Theatres (RCTs—called BRCTs in this book) in his book offered a pragmatic approach for me to view data in the context of absolute risk and to convey that data to my patients in a format that they could both understand and find relevant. I have used the BRCTs that are in that book, and have devised some of my own. I also use the BRCT concept verbally, telling my patients that in a theater of a thousand people their risk will occupy a certain number of seats that I extrapolate from available data.

I did have two criticisms of Erik's first book, which we have remedied in this version. The first is that there were simply not enough tests and procedures presented. The second is that there were no theaters showing the negative consequences of tests/treatments, especially in regard to false positives and negatives. The BRCT concept does facilitate the ability of doctors and their patients to have constructive and meaningful discussions about many medical issues in a way that is mutually satisfactory and that does not utilize excessive amounts of physician time.

The Abyss of Uncertainty

There is very little in medical care that is certain. The use of relative risks and benefits can amplify very subtle differences into what seems to be absolute certainty and can obscure an intervention's potential harms. Uncertainty is further amplified by the fickle nature of medical information. To offer an example, I recently gave a talk about the utility of supplements (vitamins, minerals), and discussed several studies that suggest Vitamin E can be dangerous without offering any benefit. The very next day, I picked up the paper and found that a new study had just been published demonstrating the utility of Vitamin E in Alzheimer's patients at doses that previous studies had declared will increase the death rate.

There is no medical certainty; studies often refute prior studies, which are then subsequently refuted by newer studies. Patients and physicians are often left in a quagmire. The populations of many studies are heavily screened, with subjects excluded if they are on certain medicines or have particular medical conditions, and thus the studies' conclusions are often not fully applicable to every patient, which explains some of their variation.

When a study focuses on a certain benefit or complication, it may obscure other benefits or risks that may be important in a patient's decision as to whether to accept the intervention. Estrogen provides a good example of this. During my early years of doctoring most physicians understood the value of estrogen in post-menopausal women, with ample studies using relative risk numbers to demonstrate the hormone's benefit in cardiac disease, bone density, and even longevity. Then the Women's Health Study repudiated many benefits of estrogen, again using relative risk to show that estrogen is actually very dangerous to women.

Now virtually no doctor will prescribe estrogen, nor will most of my patients dare take it. But are the risks of estrogen in absolute terms severe enough to warrant such a guttural reaction? Are those risks applicable to every patient, or will some perhaps benefit from estrogen, especially those without a uterus who will not have to also take progesterone? Does estrogen provide other positive effects—fewer hot flashes, less fatigue, fewer fractures, better muscle strength—that a patient may desire despite what risks estrogen may convey? In order to initiate a dialogue about such important issues, it is vital that both doctor and patient start with accurate and easily understood risk/benefit numbers. The BRCTs have provided me with that information, so that instead of using often misleading relative risk numbers from multiple conflicting studies, we can start our conversation with a range of absolute risks and benefits that will be more constructive in taking the next steps in our decision making process. To use the estrogen example, many patients, after learning about the true extent of their risk through BRCTs, something I try to extrapolate to their particular circumstances, choose to use the drug despite those risks because of other benefits they may derive. Decision making between patient and doctor is much more satisfying to both using this model.

Another use of BRCTs in my practice is in distinguishing between statistical and clinical benefit of certain interventions. For example, statin cholesterol medicines will clearly reduce cholesterol levels, so if improving the cholesterol number is the measure of the drug's success, than the entire theater will fill up in a statin BRCT. But if the outcome we want to measure is a statin's impact on death, heart attack, or stroke—all of which are clinically significant outcomes—then the theater may be more nuanced. And if we juxtapose the benefits of statins with possible risks, something that can also be presented in a BRCT model, then a more balanced assessment can begin. All those are possible with a visual display of absolute risk and benefits that focus on relevant clinical outcomes. At my recent talk about supplements someone asked me if Cheerios can decrease cholesterol, as the advertisements claim. Yes, I said, but the drop in cholesterol does not correlate with any reduction in heart disease or death, and so the chairs in a Cheerio's theater measuring clinical benefit would be empty.

Sensible Assessments Made Easy

When I discuss a test or procedure with a patient I ask several questions that help us determine its utility. First, what are we looking for? No test should be done to merely fish for problems; every test should have a specified purpose. Second, is what we are looking for amenable to treatment, what are the side effects of treatment, and is the treatment something that the patient is willing to accept? Third, what are the consequences of not doing the test? In other words, will the test reveal a condition that, if not treated, will cause harm? And fourth, what are the risks of doing the test? These questions can be answered directly from the BRCT.

Mammograms, which we discuss in this book, are illustrative of how the process may work. When we discuss mammograms, the first question is answered fairly simply: we are looking for breast cancer. As for the second question, many of my older patients would not want any treatment for breast cancer if it is found, and thus we would not necessarily conduct the test for them. But if a patient would accept treatment, then we move on to the third question, which asks what the risk is of not doing the mammogram. To merely state that mammograms can lead to a 30 % drop in breast cancer death is not helpful in ascertaining risk. Rather, using a theatrical presentation showing that 0–2 patients out of a 1,000 patients screened can avert breast cancer death if they get a mammogram will provide my patient concrete information to show the risk of not doing the test: That approximately 1 out of a 1,000 of them will die of breast cancer by not getting a mammogram. Another theater showing the risks of mammography (false positive tests that can lead to unnecessary biopsies and treatment) can help delineate if the test can cause harm. The data can then be personalized to be more applicable to my patient. For instance my older patients likely will have a lower risk of dying of breast cancer, and will thus have closer to 0–1 seats in the lives saved BRCT, while my patients with a strong family history of breast cancer may have more seats. Similarly, my patients with cystic breasts will have a higher likelihood of false positives. Some of my patients may look at that data and think that the benefits are well worth the risks. Others, especially those who are older or who have had several false alarms in the past, may look at the benefits of screening and find them to be inconsequential, choosing not to get the mammogram. In either scenario, the BRCT provides an objective measure that helps a patient reach a sensible conclusion when juxtaposed with other considerations.

Another case that we will discuss in more depth later involves bone density screening, something recommended by both Medicare through its quality control initiative and by the ACA through its Accountable Care Organizations. The purpose of bone density screening is to determine if women are at risk for osteoporosis (thinning of the bones) and thus for bone fractures. The latter measure is the only clinically relevant outcome about which doctor and patient should be concerned. Thus, the first question as to why we are doing the test is to prevent fracture, not to merely measure bone density. The second question asks if a screened patient found to be at a higher risk of fracture would accept treatment. The primary treatment of osteoporosis is a class of medicines call bisphosphonates. Many of my patients have either been intolerant of bisphosphonates, have medical conditions that prevent them from using bisphosphonates, or simply do not want to take them. If that is the case, then there is no good reason to do the test. Finally, it is necessary for any patient who is willing to accept treatment to know how good bisphosphonates are at preventing bone fractures and how frequently they induce side effects. These facts can be best presented through BRCTs.

A Patient-Centered Approach

Ultimately engaging in a rational risk assessment is satisfying for both doctors and patients and, when done with a BRCT model, does not have to utilize excessive amounts of office time. When we live in a medical environment saturated by tests, drugs, and procedures, and when we live in a world when outcomes are distorted by relative numbers that exaggerate the risks and benefits of everything, we need a more sensible way to determine which interventions are most appropriate for our patients. For me, the BRCTs are a door to a better approach.

I have used BRCT scenarios for the past several years to discuss everything from stress tests to smoking cessation to the use of calcium. With absolute risk data presented to them as part of a more general discussion, my patients have been put in the role of decision makers and directors of their own health, while I serve as their guide. Each of my patients makes unique choices based on his or her individual risk, preferences, and outlooks. But what is most important is that they do make their own decisions, and they relish the opportunity to do so.

I am excited to be part of a book that expands the BRCT concept and creates new and more effective tools that make patient-centered medicine easy for all physicians and patients to utilize. It is not beneficial for either doctor or patient to be swayed by the sensationalism to which we are exposed incessantly, and that drives our decision making in directions that are not sensible. Nor is it helpful to simply have the doctor dictate a plan without involving the patient in the discussion. A patient-centered approach need not be time consuming or contentious if done well. We hope that this book helps initiate a pragmatic means of accomplishing a very satisfying outcome.

Chapter 5
BRCTs

The core of this book consists of case studies on screening tests, drugs, surgeries, and other forms of medical intervention. We have not conducted any of the research referenced in this book. We have used a unique graphic to present, in absolute terms, findings from recent, independent, robust studies. We believe our approach will encourage each patient to determine her/his level of individual acceptable risk. We also believe our paradigm represents a much improved decision aid, with the potential for universal applicability. Due to its importance, significance, and notoriety, we have selected breast cancer screening to illustrate why our approach may be of interest to the medical community and patients.

Recently, reports on the benefits and risks of mammograms have flooded the media. In articles, Op-Ed pieces and letters to the editor, prominent representatives from the medical community and articulate members of the public have eloquently expressed their views and perspectives on this subject. Some of these commentaries are diametrically opposed to screening—others fully embrace and support the use of mammograms, and some conclude there is too much uncertainty to make an evidence-based decision.

What is certain, however, is that the current attention given to mammograms will dissipate and women in the US and throughout the world will not be any closer to making an informed choice regarding what constitutes an acceptable level of individual risk. Why is this happening? Why are medical experts, in vitriolic terms, talking past each other? Why are women becoming more apprehensive and anxious rather than becoming empowered?

It is time to answer these questions if patients are going to meaningfully participate in decisions regarding the use of mammograms and many other medical tests and treatments. It needs to be acknowledged that many patients want to be in a position to make the final decision regarding medical intervention—such as whether to be screened for breast cancer.

A typical example of this seemingly endless problem can be found in a recent article in the NYT (*Vast Study Casts Doubts on Value of Mammograms*, 2/11/2014). This article focuses on the results of a large and meticulous Canadian study on the

© Springer International Publishing Switzerland 2015

E. Rifkin, A. Lazris, *Interpreting Health Benefits and Risks*,

DOI 10.1007/978-3-319-11544-3_5

benefits and risks of mammograms. The study found that the death rates from breast cancer and from all other causes were similar in women who routinely underwent mammograms and those who did not.

The statistics were presented in easily digested, absolute terms: 1 woman in 1,000 who starts screening in her 40s, 2 who start in their 50s, and 3 who start in their 60s will avoid a breast cancer death. Values presented this way are a first step to providing patients with an opportunity to evaluate their own individual acceptable risk levels based on their interpretation of the data.

But just presenting absolute numbers is unlikely to provide a woman with the ability to determine her individual acceptable risk level. The numbers have to be framed using a familiar context. Using a Breast Cancer Screening BRCT, this is how we would suggest presenting this information to a patient (Fig. 5.1).

Given the costs, inconvenience, unpleasantness, and adverse impacts of mammograms many women may look at the BRCT and decide to forgo breast cancer screening, especially given the high false positive rate of mammograms. For example, among a thousand 50-year-old American women screened annually for a decade, 490–670 will have at least 1 false alarm and 3–14 will be over diagnosed and treated needlessly. If this information were provided to women in a BRCT format, it would serve as an objective framework to assess and compare the risks of mammograms with the absolute survival advantage of having the test (see Chap. 6 on Mammograms).

As previously discussed, unfortunately, absolute numbers are rarely used by the press and medical community to characterize the risks and benefits of mammograms and, as mentioned earlier, another statistical method (relative risks) is now routinely used to convey health risk and benefit information to the public. Case in point—in the same New York Times exchange mentioned above, Dr. Richard C. Wender, chief of cancer control for the American Cancer Society, used the relative risk approach when asked about the study's findings, "… combined data from clinical trials of mammography showed it reduces the death rate from breast cancer by at least 15 % for women in their 40s and by at least 20 % for older women." When compared with 1 in a 1,000, 15–20 % makes it appear as though mammograms significantly reduce the incidence of breast cancer deaths. But what does 15–20 % really mean?

One in 1,000 is something we can get our arms around—One person out of 1,000 benefits. We can picture ourselves in a theater with 1,000 other people and estimate the odds of our being the 1 person benefiting. But how does one assess the importance of reducing a death rate by 20 %? There is no context within which a reasonable decision can be made. What if mammograms reduce death from 2/1000 to 1/1000? That is 50 % reduction in death. Despite its seemingly impressive significance, 15–20 % could, and usually does, constitute a very small benefit, as it does in the case of mammograms.

This is not a small technical point we are making. This problem is both serious and pervasive, and it drives a great deal of confusion and unnecessary, costly and potentially risky medical decisions. Given the emphasis being placed on SDM and the importance of communication between patients and doctors, more emphasis should be placed on the appropriate way to present findings to the public.

Benefits of Breast Cancer Screening (Mammograms)

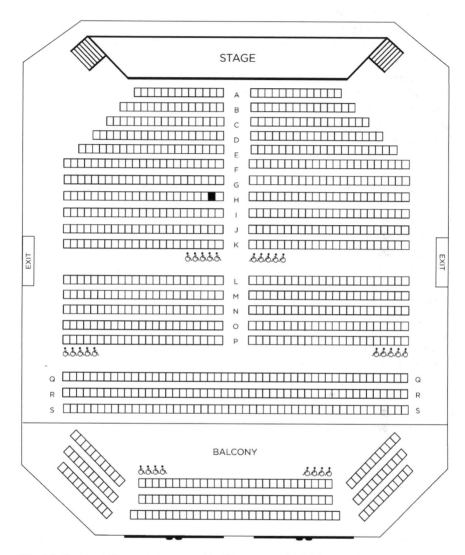

Fig. 5.1 Benefits of breast cancer screening (Mammograms). If there were 1,000 women sitting in a theater who never had a mammogram over a lifetime, there will be approximately one additional death, represented by one blackened seat, over that time period, when compared to 1,000 women who did undergo screening over a lifetime

We need to reach a point where doctors, politicians, insurance companies, medical journals, and government agencies demand that information be presented in ways that encourage patients to become more involved in decision making. A woman contemplating having periodic mammograms should request absolute benefit and risk values from her doctor in order to make an informed decision.

The following chapters consist of 19 case studies that include BRCTs for well-known screening tests, drugs, surgeries, and other types of medical intervention. Each chapter has a consistent format. They begin with a brief "story" which sets the stage; key questions presented in bullet form; risks and benefits presented in bullet form as well; and relevant BRCTs. All of this information is stated in an easily digested format that enables doctors and patients to share material when addressing risks and benefits from medical intervention. The next section of each chapter, the discussion, is more technical and was written using medical terms and concepts more familiar to physicians. The last section contains references so that our sources for information contained in the BRCTs are readily available.

In this book, we have translated confusing statistics into meaningful absolute values that doctors and patients can mutually utilize to help guide decisions. By using our graphics, conversations about important medical tests and treatment can occur during an office visit in a time efficient and useful way. We hope this is a first step toward a more broad utilization of absolute-value decision aids in the health care industry.

Part II
Case Studies: Health Benefits and Risks

Chapter 6
Breast Cancer Screening: Mammograms

Mrs. M questioned whether she should get another mammogram. She was in her upper 50s, and thus clearly within the age group where mammograms are not only recommended but have also been demonstrated to reduce breast cancer mortality. Her friends and family wanted her to get the test, and everything she read insisted she get her mammogram every year. Even her insurance company and the mammogram facility sent her reminders to assure that she get her annual screening.

"It's such an easy test," she told me, "but I hate it."

I asked her why she felt compelled to get the test, and why her family was pushing her in that direction.

"That's easy," she said. "Everyone knows that it saves lives. I heard it cuts the risk of dying in half. Really, I would have to be crazy not to get it."

I then asked her why she was reluctant to get the test.

"It hurts," she said with a smile. "You should try it once and see what it feels like. And the last two times I had it they found abnormal stuff. I had to get an ultrasound and another kind of mammogram, and then had to go for a biopsy to prove it wasn't cancer. That's the third biopsy I had to have. My sister and mother went through the same thing."

She admitted to being very anxious after every mammogram, losing sleep, and even missing days of work. She was having panic attacks simply thinking about getting the test again.

Mrs. M knew a friend who had a breast cancer discovered with a mammogram and she was treated and cured. She also knew of several people who died from breast cancer, and they had been getting mammograms too. So to her, despite everything she heard and was told, she was not convinced that mammograms were really helping to keep people alive longer. And she knew that for her, there did not seem to be any sense in finding more false positives and having more biopsies that revealed nothing. She seemed very torn about what to do.

We talked about what the likelihood was that a mammogram could prevent a breast cancer death, and what the likelihood was that a mammogram would show

E. Rifkin, A. Lazris, *Interpreting Health Benefits and Risks*, DOI 10.1007/978-3-319-11544-3_6

another false positive finding that would potentially require more testing or a biopsy. Mrs. M looked at the numbers and, without a pause, declared that she was done getting mammograms. Others of my patients look at those same numbers and come to the opposite conclusion, but for Mrs. M, whose anxiety level escalated when even discussing breast cancer screening given her past experience, the numbers actually helped to allay her fears.

A. Key Questions

- Given a patient's personal demographics and family history, how good is mammography at detecting a cancer that, if not removed, would be potentially dangerous?
- What are the personal risks of mammography? What is the likelihood that a mammogram will detect a finding that is not cancer but requires further testing?
- What are the next steps typically taken if the mammogram is abnormal, and would the patient be willing to undergo those steps?
- If breast cancer is detected, would the patient accept treatment? What are typical treatments?
- If the patient agrees to mammography, how often should it be done? If done less than the recommended rate, how will that impact her health?
- At what age should patients stop getting mammograms?

B. Risks and Benefits

- Mammography has become an accepted screening procedure that is sanctioned by most cancer organizations and is paid for annually by most insurance carriers. Women typically start screening at age 45 and continue to have the test annually for much of their lives. New recommendations suggest that screening stop in the mid-70s.
- **The most recent studies suggest that, with lifetime screening, approximately 1/1,000 breast cancer deaths are averted compared to those who are not screened (Fig. 6.1).**
- There is little empirical evidence that the overall death rate is decreased with mammograms.
- Mammograms do have a large false positive rate, with over 500/1,000 women screened having abnormalities on their mammogram that are later found to be benign. One recent study suggested that 200/1,000 women screened develop psychological trauma from the high rate of abnormal mammograms, **while 64/1,000 women screened have unnecessary biopsies (Fig. 6.2).**
- **Of 1,000 screened with mammograms over a lifetime, 10 have unnecessary treatment, which includes 2.4/1,000 who have unnecessary surgery, radiation, or chemotherapy (Fig. 6.3).**

BRCTs:
Breast Cancer Screening: Mammograms

Benefits of Breast Cancer Screening

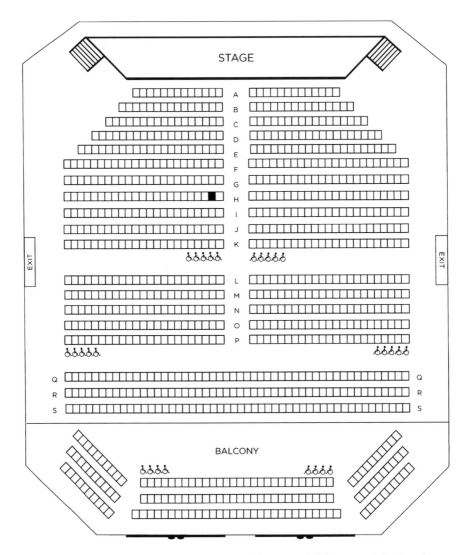

Fig. 6.1 Breast cancer screening: mammograms. If there were 1,000 women sitting in a theater who have had mammograms over a lifetime, there would be approximately 1 less breast cancer death, represented by 1 blackened seat, over that time period when compared to 1,000 women who have not had mammograms

Frequency of False Positives in Abnormal Mammograms

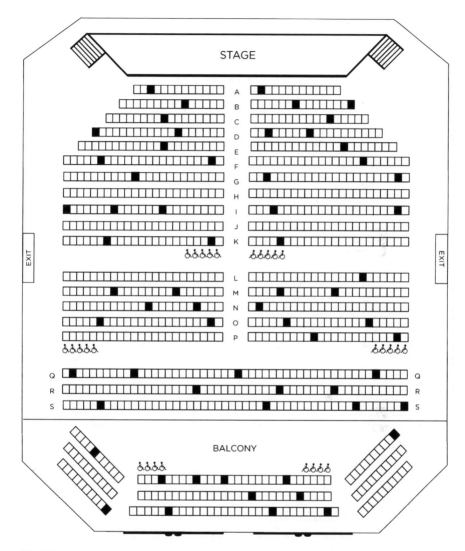

Fig. 6.2 Frequency of false positives in abnormal mammograms. If there were 1,000 women sitting in a theater who have had mammograms over a lifetime, there would be an additional 64 women, represented by blackened seats, who require a biopsy for what proves to be a benign lesion compared to 1,000 women not screened. Overall with mammography, 500 out of 1,000 women have false positive results compared to those who did not undergo screening

Unnecessary Treatment as a Result of Mammograms

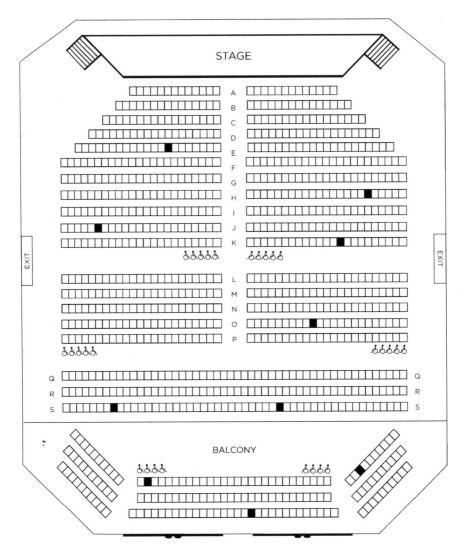

Fig. 6.3 Unnecessary treatment as a result of mammograms. If there were 1,000 women sitting in a theater who have had mammograms over a lifetime, ten additional women, represented by blackened seats, would be subjected to unnecessary treatment when compared to 1,000 women who did not undergo screening. This includes an excess of 2.4 people out of 1,000 who have unnecessary surgery, radiation, or chemotherapy

C. Discussion

The primary purpose of screening mammography is to detect breast cancer at its earliest stage so that it can be effectively treated. Breast cancer is a prevalent and devastating disease in women. The lifetime risk of developing breast cancer in American women is about 120/1,000, and approximately 40,000 people die of breast cancer each year. This risk decreases after the age of 60.[1,2] The risk is higher with people who have a strong family history and who carry a certain genetic mutation. Breast cancer can lead to death even decades after it is initially discovered.

Since breast cancers often do metastasize, especially in younger women, it is felt that waiting for a cancer to form a palpable lump is often too late. Mammograms can detect abnormal clusters of calcium in the breast that are harbingers of either cancer or carcinoma-in-situ, which is believed will transform into cancer if left alone. An early study suggests that in 3 years approximately 50/1,000 indeterminate micro-calcifications transform into cancer [1]. The sensitivity and specificity of micro-calcifications are low. Approximately 10–20/1,000 breast cancers produce micro-calcifications, and approximately 10–20/1,000 micro-calcifications become cancer.[3] Therefore, the presence or absence of these calcifications does not indicate that a person either has or is free from cancer.

After an abnormal mammogram, patients will often be biopsied with a needle to extract tissue and ascertain whether the area of concern is cancerous. Depending on that result, patients may elect to have the breast removed (mastectomy), have the cancer removed from the breast followed by 6 weeks of daily radiation treatments (lumpectomy), receive hormonal treatments, and/or even receive chemotherapy.

Do mammograms mitigate the risk of dying from breast cancer? The US Preventive Service Task Force recommends mammogram screening every other year for women between 50 and 75 years old. The data for screening under 50 is specious and individualized, and, according to the site, "Among women 75 years and older, evidence of benefits of mammography is lacking."[4] But what is the absolute risk reduction of mammogram screening among the 50–75 year group, which is where Mrs. M sits, and what are the risks of the test itself?

A recent, robust study suggests that among 1,000 women screened with mammograms, one cancer death may be prevented with essentially, no reduction in overall death rate. The study also suggests that over the past 30 years 1.3 million women were over-diagnosed by mammography, resulting in 64 unnecessary biopsies out of 1,000 women screened. Most tumors detected over the 30-year period, the study concluded, were not clinically relevant [2].

---

[1] http://www.cancer.gov/cancertopics/factsheet/detection/probability-breast-cancer.

[2] http://www.cancer.org/cancer/breastcancer/detailedguide/breast-cancer-key-statistics.

[3] http://www.uspreventiveservicestaskforce.org/uspstf/uspsbrca.htm.

[4] http://lubbockonline.com/business-focus/2011-10-24/microcalcifications-found-mammogram-can-lead-diagnosis-dcis-early-breast.

Several other studies have reached similar conclusions, demonstrating both minimal benefit and risk from breast cancer screening [3–6]. In the elderly, mammography leads to the detection of fewer episodes of clinically significant breast cancer and more false positive tests that cause potential harm [7]. A 2011 Cochrane analysis estimates that for every 2,000 women screened with mammography over 10 years, one will have her life prolonged, ten will receive unnecessary treatment, and 200 will experience psychological distress from false positive findings [8].

Gilbert Welch from Dartmouth, whose group has extensively studied mammograms, summarized recent findings in the *New York Times*. He reported that among 1,000 women screened with mammography, 0–3 will avoid a breast cancer death, 3–14 will be over-diagnosed and over-treated, and 490–670 will have false positive tests [9].

A recent study finds that because so many breast cancers grow slowly, do not grow at all, or actually regress, early detection of breast cancer by mammography causes 2.36/1,000 screened women to receive unnecessary and potentially dangerous surgery, chemotherapy, and/or radiation for cancers that would not have killed them [10]. This study attracted a great deal of media attention, but it seems to mirror the findings of earlier research.

A less discussed potential downside of mammography, especially with its high false positive rate leading to large numbers of biopsies and unnecessary treatments, is that people like Mrs. M become very anxious. Studies do demonstrate that many women have heightened levels of anxiety from mammograms, especially those who have several false positives [11]. Overall, women who do have mammograms should be made aware of the potential risks and benefits of the test and be prepared for the high possibility of false positives.

References

1. Berend, M., et al. (1992). The natural history of mammographic calcifications subjected to interval follow-up. *Archives of Surgery, 127*(11), 1309–1313.
2. Bleyer, A., & Welch, G. (2005). Effect of three decades of screening mammograms on breast cancer incidence. *New England Journal of Medicine, 2012*(367), 1998–2005.
3. Welch, H. G. (2009). Over diagnosis of mammogram screening: The question if not whether but how often it occurs. *British Medical Journal, 2009*(339), 182–183.
4. Welch, H. G., et al. (2010). Screening mammography: A long run for a short ride. *New England Journal of Medicine, 2010*, 363.
5. Phillips, K. A., et al. (1999). Putting the risk of breast cancer into perspective. *New England Journal of Medicine, 340*(2), 141–144.
6. Zahl, D. H., et al. (2008). The natural history of invasive breast cancer detected by screening mammography. *Archives of Internal Medicine, 168*(21), 2311–2315.
7. Smith-Bindman, R., et al. (2000). Is screening mammography effective in elderly women? *American Journal of Medicine, 108*(2), 112–119.
8. Gøtzsche, P. C., & Nielsen, M. (2011). Screening for breast cancer with mammography. *Cochrane Database of Systematic Reviews, 19*(1), CD001877.
9. Welch, H. (2013). *Breast cancer screenings: What we still don't know*. The New York Times

10. Kolata, G. (2014). *Vast study casts doubts on value of mammogram.* The New York Times, February 12, 2014. http://www.nytimes.com/2014/02/12/health/study-adds-new-doubts-about-value-of-mammograms.html?_r=0.
11. Lerman, C., et al. (1991). Psychological and behavior implications of abnormal mammograms. *Annals of Internal Medicine, 114*(8), 657–661.

Chapter 7
Colon Cancer Screening with Colonoscopy

During hospital rounds, I visited a patient who had been released from the Intensive Care Unit early that morning. Her medical condition had stabilized and in a few days she would be going home. But upon seeing me, she was irate.

Mrs. K, who was in her late 70s and in good health, had gone in for a routine colonoscopy. Soon after the procedure she developed abdominal pain and then shaking chills, causing her to go to the hospital, where she was diagnosed with a colonic perforation. Apparently the scope had punctured her colon, causing a life threatening rupture. The surgeons operated on her immediately cutting her colon in two, attaching the top part to a bag that now sat on her abdomen emptying her feces. She was put on IV antibiotics and stabilized in the ICU. Now she sat in front of me.

She tossed a few questions on my lap. How long would she need this bag to empty her bowel movements, and how would her bowel be put back together? What happens if the bag fell off? Why was she having so much gas and diarrhea? But then she hit me with really the only thing that occupied her mind: why did she have the colonoscopy in the first place?

I talked to her about the need to screen people for colon cancer, one of the most preventable cancers if found early. I even told her that I knew of several patients in which polyps were discovered that may have become cancer if left alone.

"How do you know they would have become cancers?" she asked me. "Maybe they just would have sat there and minded their own business." And then she said to me, "I wish they actually found some polyps, to be honest. They told me my colon was pristine; not a single problem. It doesn't feel that good to have to go through all this and to find out that my test was completely normal. It was totally unnecessary."

Well, I told her, you never know until you do the test.

"I had no symptoms," she said. "Normal bowel movements every day. I felt good. All my labs were ok. I just don't know why I said yes to the test. I was told it's time to get a colonoscopy, and so I just did it. If I knew this could happen, I would have just said no."

© Springer International Publishing Switzerland 2015
E. Rifkin, A. Lazris, *Interpreting Health Benefits and Risks*,
DOI 10.1007/978-3-319-11544-3_7

Recently I gave a talk on bowel health to a group of elderly residents of a retirement community. I relayed the story of Mrs. K, only to emphasize that it is important to assess the risks and benefits of every test and to make a rational decision before agreeing. At the end of the talk one person, who looked to be in her 80s, said she was scheduled for a colonoscopy but now planned to cancel it. I did not want my talk to impact her decision, since there were certainly benefits of colon evaluations in many circumstances. But she had made up her mind; she never wanted the test and felt it was forced upon her. After hearing about the actual data, she now felt she could say no.

A. Key Questions

- At what ages are colonoscopies most effective in preventing colon cancer?
- Do all colon polyps transform into cancer if left alone? What is the chance that the polyps that are discovered and removed by colonoscopy would have become cancerous?
- What is the absolute risk reduction with colonoscopy screening for colon cancer and death over a person's lifetime?
- What is the potential harm of getting a colonoscopy?
- Do we have information about how often people should get colonoscopies?

B. Risks and Benefits

- Colon cancer is one of the leading causes of cancer death in this country, and many people who develop colon cancer have no symptoms. Approximately, 950/1,000 cancers occur after the age of 50. Colonoscopy screening in asymptomatic patients can detect polyps that can transform into cancer and thus help prevent colon cancer. It is felt that after age 75 the risk of colonoscopy exceeds any lifetime benefit, although precise numbers are not available.
- Approximately 920/1,000 high-grade polyps do not progress to cancer over the typical 10-year interval between colon screenings. Therefore, the vast majority of polyps removed confer no risk.
- **Large studies have demonstrated that 1.5–3 colon cancer deaths are averted over 10 years for every 1,000 people screened (Fig. 7.1).**
- **The risk of severe complications from colonoscopy, including perforation, hospitalization, and death, is approximately 2.5/1,000 people screened, and that number increases with age (Fig. 7.2).**
- There is no reliable data suggesting what the optimal time period should be between colonoscopy screenings. Since the reduction in colon cancer deaths is 0.15–0.3/1,000 people screened per year, and since the complication rate rises with age, a patient's overall life expectancy can help determine if colonoscopy screening is more likely to cause harm than benefit.

BRCTs:
Colon Cancer Screening with Colonoscopy

Effectiveness of Colonoscopies in Preventing Colon Cancer Death

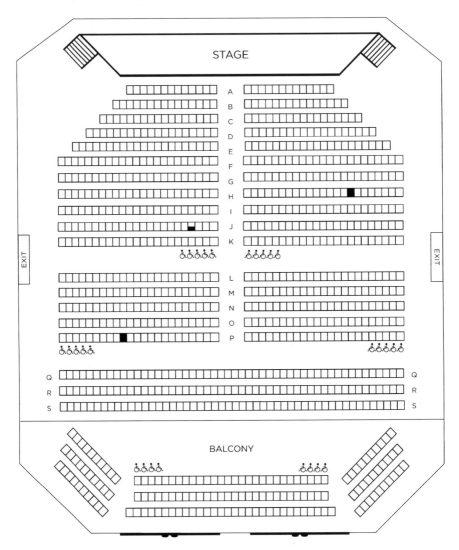

Fig. 7.1 Effectiveness of colonoscopies in preventing colon cancer death. Out of 1,000 asymptomatic people sitting in a theater who have been screened with colonoscopy, 1.5–3 colon cancer deaths, represented by blackened seats, will be averted over 10 years compared to 1,000 people who are not screened. There is no overall reduction in total death rate

Major Complications from Colonoscopies

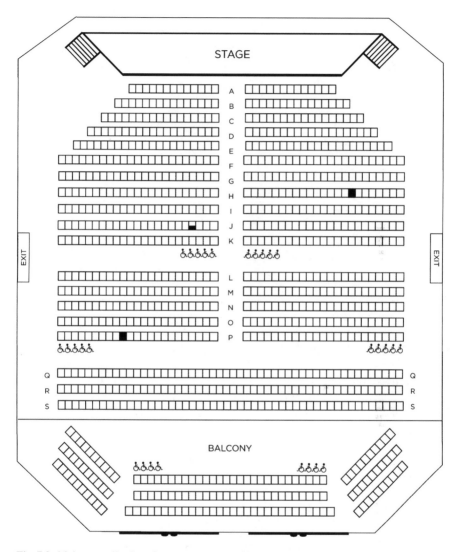

Fig. 7.2 Major complications from colonoscopies. Out of 1,000 asymptomatic people sitting in a theater who are screened with colonoscopy, 2.5 of them, represented by blackened seats, will have major complications, such as bowel perforation, at the time of surgery. That number increases as people age

C. Discussion

In this country over 140,000 people are diagnosed with and 50,000 people die from colon cancer annually. Approximately, 950/1,000 colon cancer deaths occur after the age of 50. Recently the incidence of colon cancer mortality has been steadily falling, something that has been ascribed to a very deliberate screening effort to find pre-cancerous polyps and remove them before they become malignant.[1] Some patients exhibit worrisome signs that could portend the presence of colon polyps or cancer, such as rectal bleeding, new anemia, weight loss, change in bowel habits, or abdominal pain. Other people are at high risk for colon cancer, especially those with a strong family history, those who smoke, and those who are obese.

Most cancers, though, develop before symptoms occur and not in high risk people. For this reason, the preponderance of cancer organizations recommends screening for colon cancer in asymptomatic patients at regular intervals. The primary goal of screening is to find and remove polyps before they either trigger symptoms or transform into cancer, and the main instrument employed to accomplish that goal is a colonoscopy. Colon polyps are more prevalent as people age, and the primary fear of allowing them to grow is that some of them can transform into cancer. One study showed that 80/1,000 high risk polyps progress to cancer over 10 years [1]. It is felt that removing polyps will thus prevent them from becoming cancerous. However, since 920/1,000 polyps will not transform into cancer over a 10-year period, the false positive rate of polyp detection and removal is 920/1,000.

Colonoscopies are not without risk. Patients must endure a "prep" that is both burdensome and potentially dangerous. They typically undergo anesthesiology during the procedure, which carries potential risk. Colonoscopies can also puncture the colon, instigate bleeding, and even lead to death. The rates of these complications must be weighed against the cancer-averting benefits that colonoscopies confer. For patients, especially those who are told that they must have colonoscopies every 3–10 years depending on their circumstances, it is important to know the absolute risks and benefits of the procedure.

The US Preventive Services Task Force (USPSTF) recommends colon cancer screening from age 50 to 75. After age 75 the risks of screening outweigh the benefits given the co-morbidities of that age group. Before age 50 there is a low likelihood of finding polyps, and thus the risks also outweigh the benefits. But what are the potential benefits and risks?[2]

A recent *New England Journal of Medicine* study[3] followed 2,600 people who had colonoscopy and polyp removal over a 20-year interval and compared them to a similar population who had not had colon cancer screening. The study was not

---

[1] http://www.cancer.org/acs/groups/content/@epidemiologysurveilance/documents/document/acspc-028323.pdf.

[2] http://www.uspreventiveservicestaskforce.org/uspstf/uspscolo.htm.

[3] http://www.nytimes.com/2012/02/23/health/colonoscopy-prevents-cancer-deaths-study-finds.html?pagewanted=all&_r=0.

randomized, and subjects were given routine colonoscopies for colon screening only if they were in the target group. The death rate from colon cancer for the screened group was 12 deaths vs. 25 expected deaths in the non-screened group, which translates to five lives from colon cancer saved out of 1,000 people screened over approximately 16 years, or 3.125 lives saved/1,000 screenings over 10 years, which is the typical interval between screenings [2].

A more recent analysis followed 89,000 people over 22 years from the nurses' health study and the health professional study, comparing those who were screened with colonoscopy and those who were not. Overall there were 474 colon cancer deaths in the group over that time frame. There were three cancer deaths/1,000 people in the non-screened group and 1.5 deaths/1,000 in the colonoscopy group, for a final result of 1.5 colon cancer deaths prevented/1,000 people receiving colonoscopy over 10 years [3]. Several previous studies do not show any change in all-cause mortality, [4] meaning that with screening people may not live any longer.

The USPSTF cites the risk of perforation with a colonoscopy as being 0.38/1,000 people screened. The risk of serious complications that likely will require hospitalization, including perforation and infection, is cited to be 2.5/1,000 people screened in a year. Mrs. K's perforation would fall into the latter category and was considered life threatening. There was no way to ascertain if she would be at high risk for serious complications by an exam or pre-test evaluation, although by USPSTF standards she was too old to benefit from screening and was at an age where colonoscopy risk is deemed to be high. The risk of perforation and serious complications increases with age, and the benefits of screening diminish,[4,5] which is why the USPSTF advises that screening stop well before Mrs. K's age.

References

1. Strykes, S., et al. (1987). Natural history of untreated colonic polyps. *Gastroenterology, 93*(5), 1009–1013.
2. Zauber, A. G., et al. (2012). Colonoscopic polypectomy and long-term prevention of colorectal cancer deaths. *New England Journal of Medicine, 366,* 687–696.
3. Nishihara, R., et al. (2013). Long-term colorectal cancer incidence and mortality after lower endoscopy. *New England Journal of Medicine, 369*(12), 1095–1105.
4. Hadler, N. M. (2009). *The last well person* (pp. 71–72). Montreal: McGill-Queen's University Press.

---

[4] http://newoldage.blogs.nytimes.com/2013/03/12/too-many-colonoscopies-in-the-elderly/.

[5] http://www.ncbi.nlm.nih.gov/pmc/articles/PMC2917147/.

Chapter 8
Prostate Cancer Screening

Mr. M came in to talk to me about his PSA (prostate-specific antigen). At age 67 he already had learned far too much about this simple blood test used to detect prostate cancer. His had been slightly elevated for many years, followed closely by an urologist. His urologist checked it fairly regularly, but when it rose to about four he talked Mr. M into getting a biopsy. Fearing the specter of prostate cancer, and incessantly stressed as he watched the PSA creep up every time it was checked, Mr. M agreed. The biopsy consisted of many needles being pushed into his gland, leading to several weeks of pain and even some transient difficulty urinating. On the positive side, the needles detected only some atypical cells, but no definitive cancer.

The urologist did a few ultrasounds on his prostate over the next few years and continued to check the PSA and a digital rectal exam twice a year. At first all had been ok. But now, over the past year, the PSA had started to climb again, now drifting up close to 10.

"It's totally stressing me out," Mr. M told me. "And the thought of going for another biopsy is driving me crazy. But that's what he wants to do. I just want your advice."

Mr. M did have a slightly enlarged prostate. He also had symptoms of BPH (benign prostate hyperplasia) including waking up twice at night to urinate and having a slow urinary stream. We talked about how the increasing size of his prostate could falsely elevate the PSA value.

"How do I know the difference between a high PSA that is from cancer and one that is just from a big prostate?"

I told him that his question was an excellent one, but not one easily answered. I showed him some data about the predictive value of PSA including the rate of false positives and the inability of PSA to determine if a person had a cancer that was potentially dangerous. I explained that many men did have prostate cancer as they aged, but fewer died of the cancer. Because he was so young, he may not want to live with prostate cancer for the next 20 years, but in fact there was no way of telling whether such cancer would be lethal or even harmful. Most were not.

© Springer International Publishing Switzerland 2015
E. Rifkin, A. Lazris, *Interpreting Health Benefits and Risks*,
DOI 10.1007/978-3-319-11544-3_8

"Even if this next biopsy shows that you have a cancer," I told him, "there is no certainty that treating that cancer will lead to improved outcome. There is a very high risk, though, that treatment will really cause you a lot of problems." Again, I showed him some data.

He mulled over it. "Don't you think that the normal biopsy I had before was enough? I mean, how likely would it be now for cancer to show up? And even if it did, wouldn't it probably be the slow kind of cancer anyway since my PSA has been high for so long?"

None of his questions had easy answers, but we did discuss the fact that a biopsy based on a PSA value could cause him harm, especially if it led to surgery or radiation treatment, with a low and uncertain absolute chance of helping him live longer or better. For now, he decided to skip the biopsy, and he said he may not even get another PSA, at least for a while. We both agreed to the plan.

A. Key Questions

- Is there evidence that PSA screening increases survival by detecting prostate cancer early?
- Is there evidence that prostate surgery results in impotence (erectile dysfunction)?
- Is there evidence that prostate surgery results in incontinence (inability to control urine)?
- What are other side effects from prostate surgery?
- Is it true that the most common kind of prostate cancer is slow growing (i.e., indolent) and does not need to be treated in most instances?
- Do prostate biopsies result in health complications?

B. Risks and Benefits of Prostate Screening

- At present, empirical data are insufficient to calculate the absolute risk for individuals who are or are not screened with PSA. Current data is anecdotal (i.e., subjective, heresy). The primary reason is that men with indolent or slow-growing prostate cancer will die of something else; therefore, there is insufficient data to determine benefits of screening.
- **Given this high level of uncertainty, we cannot find the absolute risk reduction values for screening, and we cannot compare survival benefits between the two groups. Therefore, it is not possible to construct a Prostate Cancer Screening BRCT (see Fig. 8.1).**

- On the other hand, there are significant serious risks among men who undergo prostatectomy (prostate-removal surgery for prostate cancer) and/or radiation.
- **After prostatectomy or radiation, sexual dysfunction appears more prevalent than previously reported, according to a recent comprehensive article in the National Cancer Institute Journal (NCIJ) (Fig. 8.2)**
- **In the same NCIJ article, urinary incontinence also appears to be a major problem after prostatectomy or radiation (Fig. 8.3).**
- Biopsies can have serious side effects, including bleeding and infection.

BRCTs:
Prostate Cancer Screening

Benefits from Prostate Surgery and/or Radiation

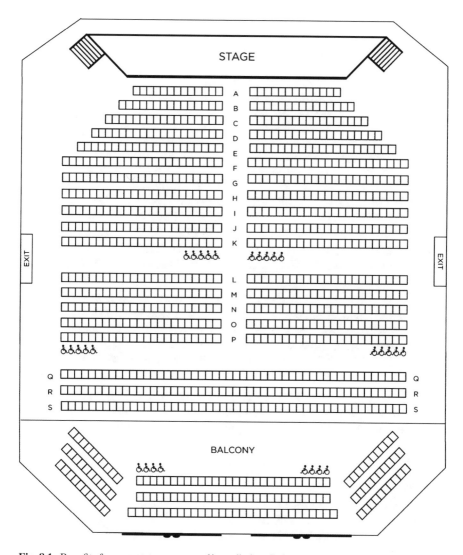

Fig. 8.1 Benefits from prostate surgery and/or radiation. Robust comprehensive studies have concluded that there is no scientific evidence that prostate screening tests have any death benefits when compared with groups who have not been screened. Therefore, this prostate BRCT contains no blackened dots

Risks of Impotence Resulting from Prostate Surgery and/or Radiation of the Prostate Gland

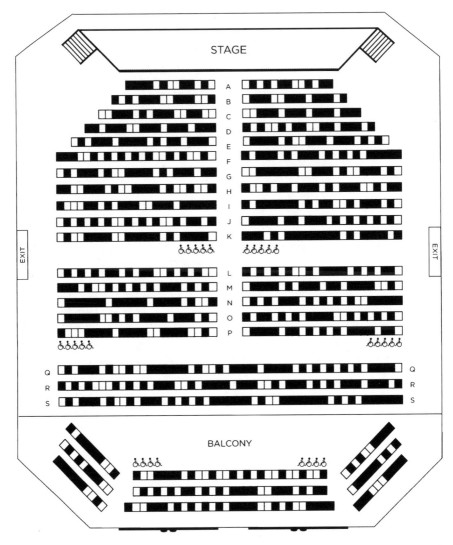

Fig. 8.2 Risks of impotence resulting from prostate surgery and/or radiation of the prostate gland. This BRCT shows the number of men (600), represented by blackened dots, out of 1,000, who became impotent after prostate surgery and/or radiation, based on recent findings in NCIJ

Risks of Incontinence Resulting from Prostate Surgery and/or Radiation of the Prostate Gland

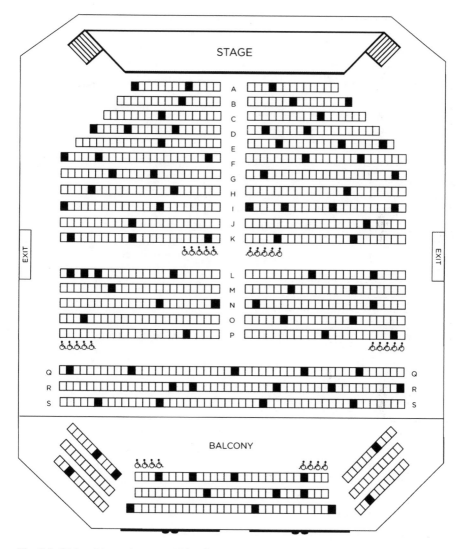

Fig. 8.3 Risks of incontinence resulting from prostate surgery and/or radiation of the prostate gland. This BRCT represents the number of men (90), represented by blackened dots, out of 1,000, who become incontinent after surgery and/or radiation, based on recent findings in NCIJ

C. Discussion

The benefit of screening for prostate cancer using prostate-specific antigen (PSA) testing and digital rectal exam (DRE) is uncertain and has been the subject of a comprehensive, randomized, prospective trial conducted by the National Cancer Institute [1]. After 13 years of follow up, men who underwent annual prostate cancer screening with PSA testing and men in the control group had the same rate of death from the disease. It should be noted that men in the control arm also had PSA screening frequently. No evidence of a mortality benefit was seen overall or in subgroups defined by age, the presence of other illnesses, or pre-trial PSA testing. However, there were harms associated with follow-ups of abnormal screening tests and with treatments.

Prostate cancer is the most frequently diagnosed solid tumor in American men. An estimated 179,300 men will be diagnosed this year (2014), and more than 70 % of these patients will have early stage, localized disease. According to the National Cancer Institute (NCI), prostate cancer is the second leading cancer killer among men [2]. An estimated one in six men will be diagnosed with prostate cancer in his lifetime, and more than 30,000 Americans die of the disease each year. As a result, the NCI and other national medical organizations emphasize the need for routine screening for prostate cancer in men over the age of 50.

Treatment options for men with tumors confined to the prostate and who have at least a 10-year life expectancy include a number of aggressive options or expectant management, also known as "watchful waiting." Each of these approaches is associated with a different spectrum of side effects that may impact quality of life in the short or long run.

Screening tests look for disease in people who do not have symptoms yet. Finding disease early can make treatment more effective, reduce suffering, and even prevent more serious problems. Screening has to be worth it: the occurrence of the disease and the chance of death must justify the effort and expense of screening [3].

Clearly, prostate cancer is common enough and serious enough to justify screening. The prostate screening test has several components. It generally involves a DRE and a blood test. If cancer is suspected, there is also a biopsy of prostate tissue. For healthy men over 50, the American Cancer Society recommends an annual DRE and blood test [1]. The blood test measures levels of a protein produced in the prostate gland called PSA. Approximately 50 % of "older men" now undergo routine PSA screenings.

There is no such thing as a normal or even abnormal PSA level. But the more PSA in his blood, the more likely it is that a man has prostate cancer. Since PSA is produced in the body and can be measured as an indicator of prostate cancer, it is sometimes called a biomarker. Several factors can cause PSA levels to fluctuate, so a single elevated PSA test does not necessarily mean anything is wrong. A high test result could be due to a harmless enlargement of the prostate, an inflammation, an infection, or even age or race. *So, even though elevated PSA is a biomarker for prostate cancer, elevated levels do not necessarily mean that there is a problem.*

Even if screening finds a tumor, the benefits of surgery are not always clear-cut. Therefore, prostate surgery does not necessarily reduce a man's chance of dying from prostate cancer. Sometimes, PSA testing finds slow-growing, indolent tumors that are unlikely to be life threatening. If and when an annual PSA test finds a fast-growing tumor, it may be too late if the aggressive cancer has already spread to other parts of the body [4].

Much is still unknown about prostate cancer. The causes are not clear. The progression of the disease from initial symptoms to death is not well-defined [4]. It seems some tumors are relatively inactive, while others progress rapidly. Prostate cancer may even be two different diseases, a faster growing one and a slower growing one.

For the more common slow-growing cancer, the time from development of the disease to the onset of symptoms is drawn-out. This long period leaves ample time to detect the indolent cancer with a screening test. But symptoms appear early in the fast-growing form, and death often follows shortly. In these cases, the asymp-tomatic stage may not be long enough to allow detection by screening. And once symptoms are evident, you know you have the disease, so there is no point in screening to look for it.

There is also a problem with false positive and false negative screening test results. False positives can occur when the PSA level is elevated even though no cancer is present.

Fortunately, most men with elevated PSA do not have cancer. Of course, it's a big relief to find out that there is no cancer after all. But the additional tests that prove the "positive" to be false have risks and cost money, not to mention the anxiety of waiting for results [5].

On the other hand, false negatives occur when prostate cancer hides behind an ordinary PSA level. Most prostate cancers are slow-growing and may exist for decades before they are large enough to cause symptoms. With a false negative, PSA results don't alert you to the problem even when the disease is significantly progressing.

PSA is just an indicator; a biopsy is needed to determine if prostate cancer is actually present. The more tissue removed during the biopsy, the greater the chance of detecting cancer. If a biopsy confirms cancer, the surgery to remove the tumor can cause incontinence and/or erectile dysfunction [4].

Reports in the news suggest that prostate cancer is often a potent, fatal disease in 50-year-old men. In fact, disease and death from prostate cancer are principally problems of older men. Age is the most common risk factor, with nearly 70 % of prostate cancer cases occurring in men aged 65 and older [6].

What does all this mean? Let's go back to the key question. Is there evidence that prostate cancer screening leads to a survival benefit due to early detection of prostate cancer? The answer is no. There is no hard evidence, only anecdotal evidence. It is possible there is a benefit, but it is also possible that screening is without any value. The data are simply insufficient to answer the question with any degree of certainty.

Considering the uncertainty, the decision to have a prostate biopsy or surgery should be weighed carefully. The fact that we cannot calculate the absolute benefits of screening calls widespread PSA screening into question. It is possible that biopsies and surgery may not be warranted. We do not mean to suggest that prostate cancer is not a deadly disease; thousands of men die from prostate cancer every year. What this case study does reveal, however, is the absence of evidence that screening tests reduce the risk of dying of this cancer. You may be willing to accept a certain level of risk from biopsies or surgery, but there is no proof that you stand to benefit.

The Prostate Cancer Outcomes Study (PCOS) [8], funded by the National Cancer Institute, is the first comprehensive, population-based assessment of sexual function and urinary continence among men treated with radical prostatectomy for early stage, localized prostate cancer. It is also the first study to examine the sexual and urinary side effects of such surgery in minority populations.

The study followed 1,291 men between the ages of 39 and 79 in six states. Sexual and urinary function was assessed, via self-administered questionnaire, at 6 months, a year, and 2 years after diagnosis (all of the men had surgery within 6 months of diagnosis). At 18 or more months after surgery, the impotence rate among these men was nearly 60 %. The majority of participants were middle-income, married, Caucasian retirees with a high-school or college education. In addition to its population-based design, the strength of the study was that it relied on self-reporting, not second-hand information.

The study also looked at the effect of the surgery on urinary control. Two years after diagnosis (at least 18 months after surgery), nearly 9 % of the participants reported that incontinence remained a "moderate to big problem," with about 40 % reporting occasional urinary leaking, 7 % complaining of frequent leaking, and 2 % having no urinary control.

Age also was significantly related to the degree and frequency of incontinence. Compared to younger men, those in their mid to late 70s experienced the highest level of incontinence; 14 % reported total incontinence 2 years after diagnosis, compared to rates ranging from less than 1 to 4 % among men under age 60. In addition, younger men regained function sooner than older men.

So what is the bottom line? The current push for prostate cancer screening has increased identification and treatment of the disease. Since the vast majority of men with prostate cancer have the indolent type and die of something else, there are insufficient data to determine the benefits of prostate cancer screening. Researchers have also found that extensive biopsies do not necessarily lead to a survival benefit due to early cancer detection [7].

Nevertheless, men often choose surgery to remove these cancers. But even without surgery, men with this slow-growing form of the disease would likely have died of heart disease, diabetes, or another form of cancer before they even developed symptoms from the prostate tumor. Therefore, even without treatment, many of these prostate cancer cases would still have been low-risk.

However, there are robust data from comprehensive studies that clearly demonstrate that the treatments themselves result in serious negative outcomes, such as impotence and incontinence, as mentioned above [8]. In assessing acceptable individual risks, men should be advised to compare and contrast the data based on absolute risks of erectile dysfunction and/ or incontinence resulting from surgery and uncertain benefits from surgery.

References

1. Andriole, G. L., Levin, D. L., Crawford, E. D., Gelmann, E. P., Pinsky, P. F., Chia, D., Kramer, B. S., Reding, D., Church, T. R., Grubb, R. L., Izmirlian, G., Ragard, L. R., Clapp, J. D., Prorok, P. C., Gohagan, J. K., & PLCO Project Team. (2005). Prostate cancer screening in the prostate, lung, colorectal and ovarian (PLCO) cancer screening trial: findings from the initial screening round of a randomized trial. *Journal of National Cancer Institute, 97*(6), 433–438.
2. Surveillance, Epidemiology, and End Results (SEER) Program (1997). Public use CD-ROM (1973–94) by the National Cancer Institute, DCPC, Surveillance Program, Cancer Statistics Branch.
3. U.S. Preventive Services Task Force. (1996). *Guide to clinical preventive services* (2nd ed.). Baltimore: Lippincott, Williams & Wilkins. 953 pp.
4. Lefevre, M. L. (1998). Prostate cancer screening: More harm than good? *American Family Physician, 58*(2), 432–438.
5. Keetch, D. W., Catalona, W. J., & Smith, D. S. (1994). Serial prostatic biopsies in men with persistently elevated serum prostate specific antigen values. *The Journal of Urology, 151*(6), 1571–1574.
6. Ries, L. A. G., Eisner, M. P., Kosary, C. L., Hanke, B. F., Miller, B. A., Clegg, L., Mariotto, A., Feuer, E. J., & Edwards, B. K. (Eds.). (2004). *SEER cancer statistics review, 1975–2001.* Bethesda, MD: National Cancer Institute. Available online at http://seer.cancer.gov/csr/1975-2001.
7. Eichler, K., Wilby, J., Hempel, S., Myers, L., & Kleijnen, J. (2005). *Diagnostic value of systematic prostate biopsy methods in the investigation for prostate cancer: A systematic review (CRD Report 29).* York: University of York. 215 pp.
8. Potosky, A. L., Davis, W. W., Hoffman, R. M., Stanford, J. L., Stephenson, R. A., Penson, D. F., & Harlan, L. C. (2014). Five-year outcomes after prostatectomy or radiotherapy for prostate cancer: The prostate cancer outcomes study. *Journal National Cancer Institute, 96*(18), 1358–1367.

Chapter 9
Screening for Lung Cancer with Spiral CT

Mr. L had been a heavy smoker much of his life. He started smoking in college and stopped at age 60, 10 years ago. At that time he was found to have a small, treatable cancer in his throat that was ascribed to his smoking. He never has had any obvious clinical ramifications from his smoking. He remained very active, without any shortness of breath or exercise limitations. He had no cough, no known lung or heart disease, and was not prone to sinus or respiratory infections. In the past several years, he has had chest x-rays for various reasons, none of which demonstrated any worrisome findings.

For many years, Mr. L expressed worry about his risk of getting lung cancer. He knew several former smokers who did get cancer even though they had been without any symptoms or worrisome signs, and all of them died. He always found excuses to get chest x-rays, even though I informed him that multiple studies showed no improved outcome in smokers screened with x-rays. In fact, as I explained to him, a normal x-ray did not rule out cancer, and a positive x-ray did not mean he had cancer and may lead to excessive and dangerous testing to rule it out. Still, every normal x-ray gave him a dose of relief. Now, he had heard from friends that a better test existed to determine if he had lung cancer, and he was interested in having me order it.

The test in question was a spiral CT scan, and a segment on the news suggested that all smokers and former heavy smokers should consider getting the test annually. In fact, it appeared that the test not only detected cancer early, but it also saved lives. Mr. L had already contacted his health insurance and learned that it would soon be covering the test to screen former smokers. He told me that getting the test was a no-brainer.

I talked about some of the dangers inherent to screening tests. These included false positive findings that might require further testing or even biopsies. I explained that in lung cancer screening the false positive rate was very high. We also discussed the ramifications of radiation exposure derived by annual CT scans, including a potentially higher risk of other cancers. I finally discussed that the CT scan study conducted

© Springer International Publishing Switzerland 2015
E. Rifkin, A. Lazris, *Interpreting Health Benefits and Risks*,
DOI 10.1007/978-3-319-11544-3_9

on smokers did not have long-term data and should probably be viewed as being preliminary in its conclusions.

But Mr. L could not see past the fact that the CT could possibly prevent a cancer death. All of the other problems I relayed to him seemed inconsequential to that fact. There was also an element of common sense ingrained in his decision-making process: how could it not be better to find a cancer as early as possible and eliminate it from the body before it caused harm? I did try to explain that some cancers never progress, some even resolve on their own, and that the diagnostic tests used to determine if nodules could be cancerous, and the treatments for cancer, could themselves cause harm.

"If you could tell me that my lungs are clear and that I won't get cancer, then I'm good with that," he said. "But if there's even a small chance of finding a cancer, even if there is some risk, I feel better doing that."

Mr. L looked at the data, and in my opinion he made a rational decision to be screened, *based on his own wishes*. We set him up for the CT scan, which in the end turned out to be normal.

A. Key Questions

- Who would most benefit from CT screening for lung cancer? What is the risk of lung cancer in smokers?
- Does spiral CT screening decrease the risk of lung cancer deaths in smokers, and by how much?
- What is the rate of false positive findings? How often would a positive CT scan result in findings that are proven not to be cancer?
- How many people undergo subsequent testing for CT findings that are non-cancerous (false positives)? What are those tests, and what are the risks of those tests?
- If a smoker is found to have a cancer, would that cancer have necessarily been lethal? Do any screened smokers have to undergo surgery for what is felt to be non-lethal cancer, and if so what is the risk of the surgery?
- Would the patient be willing and able to undergo lung biopsy? Lung surgery? What are the potential complications of such procedures?
- Do the patient's other medical conditions limit overall life expectancy in a way that would negate the advantage of lung cancer screening?

B. Risks and Benefits

- The USPSTF recommends spiral CT screening for smokers and some ex-smokers between ages 55 and 80. The lifetime excess risk of developing cancer in smokers over non-smokers is 159/1,000 for men, and 103/1,000 for women. CT screening decreases the excess cancer death rate.

- **A recent large study has demonstrated that smokers who undergo annual spiral CT screening have a 3.3/1,000 decrease in cancer death over five years (Fig. 9.1).**
- **The USPSTF cites a false positive rate of 675/1,000 in smokers receiving screening. Overall, approximately 233/1,000 smokers screened have significant false positive findings that lead to further testing. Approximately, 92/1,000 people have high-radiation PET scans and 5.8/1,000 people have lung biopsies for what prove to be non-cancerous false positives on CT scan. Lung biopsies do have a significant risk of serious complications (Fig. 9.2).** Therefore, a sizeable number of people who get CT screening and who would not die of lung cancer receive false alarms, unnecessary tests, and unnecessary procedures all of which can cause harm.
- It is estimated that of all cancers detected by CT screening and surgically removed, 180/1,000 of them are non-lethal, and if left alone would have caused no harm. Overall, 7.1/1,000 of all screened smokers have lung surgery for what is believed to be non-lethal cancer. Such surgery carries a 50/1,000 30-day risk of death, as well as many other potential complications. Therefore, many smokers who have CT detected cancers removed and who are subjected to dangerous surgery would not have died from those cancers, but may be harmed from removing the cancers.
- Since many patients would not agree to biopsy and surgery, and others have physical conditions that would render such surgery unwarranted; it is important to ascertain that information before screening is initiated. Also, many smokers have a shorter life expectancy from other smoking-related illnesses and would have dubious benefits from the detection and treatment of lung cancer.

BRCTs:
Screening for Lung Cancer with Spiral CT

Lung Cancer Deaths Averted with Annual Spiral CT Scanning

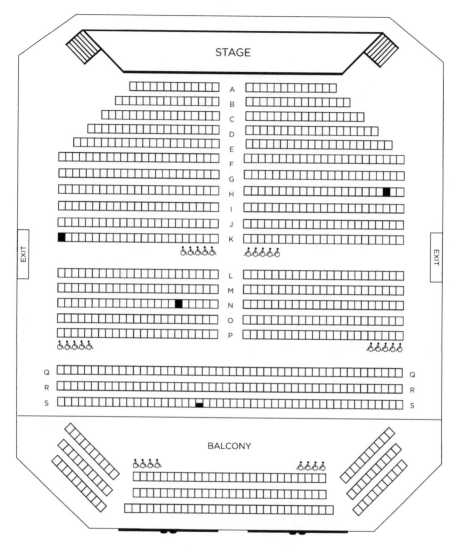

Fig. 9.1 Lung cancer deaths averted with annual spiral CT scanning. Out of 1,000 smokers or former heavy smokers in a theater who undergo annual spiral CT scans for lung cancer, 3.3, represented by blackened seats, will avoid dying of lung cancer over 5 years compared to 1,000 smokers or former heavy smokers not screened with CT scan

Harm of Yearly Spiral CT Scans for Lung Cancer

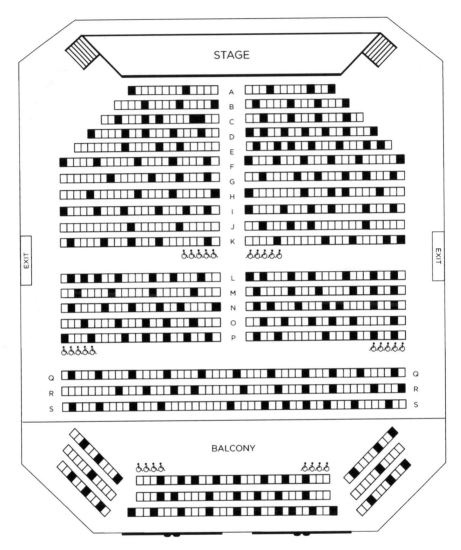

Fig. 9.2 Harm of yearly spiral CT scans for lung cancer. Out of 1,000 smokers or former heavy smokers in a theater who undergo annual spiral CT scans for lung cancer, 233, represented by blackened seats, will have persistent false positive results that lead to further testing with such modalities as PET scans or lung biopsies before they are shown not to have cancer. Overall the false positive rate for annual CT screening is 675 out of 1,000 screens

C. Discussion

Smoking is one of the leading causes of death in the world. Smokers die of heart attacks, strokes, and multiple cancers more than do non-smokers. Their life expectancy is significantly shorter. Overall smoking causes 480,000 deaths a year. Almost a half of the deaths are from cancer, a third are from vascular disease, and a quarter are from lung disease. The risk of all disease diminishes when people quit smoking, although the risk of certain cancers can linger for up to a decade.[1,2] Lung cancer is perhaps the most ominous diagnosis for smokers and is the one many fear. The lifetime risk of lung cancer among smokers is 172/1,000 for men and 116/1,000 for women, compared to 13/1,000 for non-smokers.[1]

Lung cancer is also the most lethal cancer in this country, killing more people than colon cancer, breast cancer, and prostate cancer combined. Overall, it is responsible for 160,000 cancer deaths a year, which is almost 300/1,000 of all cancer deaths in the country. The survival rate is very low for lung cancer. The overall 5-year survival is 160/1,000; over half of people diagnosed die within a year. However, when the cancers are detected early, the survival rate is much better, being closer to 500/1,000 after 5 years.[3] Certain cancers are more treatable than others. One form, called small cell cancer, is more responsive to chemotherapy and radiation than non-small cell cancer. The latter type of cancer can only be cured by surgical excision, and that is only feasible if it is detected early before it spreads. The prognosis of untreated non-small cell cancer is very poor, with a survival of approximately 7 months. It must be noted that many people with lung cancer are unable to tolerate surgery and other treatments due to smoking-related lung and heart disease [2].

Discovering lung cancers early can be problematic, since most patients do not have any symptoms. The use of chest x-ray has been controversial, since many studies have demonstrated a failure to discover cancers when they are small enough to be effectively treated. A more recent study did demonstrate that regular chest x-rays in smokers can detect more treatable lung cancers than in smokers who do not receive x-rays, but the overall death rate did not improve, and there were a large number of false positive x-rays.[4]

False positive x-rays can lead to unnecessary testing, treatment, and even death. In addition, some of the cancers detected on x-ray may never have progressed to be clinically significant. A recent study ascertained that as many as half of lung cancers found by x-ray or sputum analysis were not lethal. It was determined that those cancers, if left alone, would have led neither to harm nor death, while their detection could cause potential harm through overtreatment [3]. Also, because smokers have

---

[1] http://www.cancer.gov/cancertopics/factsheet/Tobacco/cessation.

[2] http://www.cdc.gov/tobacco/data_statistics/fact_sheets/health_effects/effects_cig_smoking/.

[3] http://www.lung.org/lung-disease/lung-cancer/resources/facts-figures/lung-cancer-fact-sheet.html.

[4] http://www.cancer.gov/newscenter/newsfromnci/2005/plcolungbaseline.

such high mortality from illnesses other than lung cancer, including heart disease and other cancers, it is questionable if finding and treating lung cancer will lead to a long-term mortality benefit.

A much more sensitive means of detecting early lung cancers is through CT scans of the lungs. Such scans have been used and studied in smokers and have produced disappointing and conflicting results [4]. CT scans also expose patients to large amounts of radiation. It is estimated that while CT scans overall comprise 30–50/1,000 of all radiologic tests, they contribute 350–450/1,000 of the total radiation exposure to patients [5]. A recent study suggested that such radiation exposure actually can cause cancer. It is estimated that from the 72 million CT scans done in 2007, 29,000 people will develop cancer, comprising 20/1,000 of all cancer diagnoses [6].

Newer CT scans can provide very detailed pictures of the lung without delivering so high a radiation dose. In spiral CT scans the radiation tube rotates around the patient, allowing the test to be conducted rapidly with one-fifth of the radiation of traditional CT scans. This is equivalent to the radiation exposure of about 15 traditional x-rays. New research has determined that spiral CT scans can potentially detect early lung cancers and improve the death rate of smokers and former smokers. Spiral CT screening is now becoming accepted by many insurance companies as a viable screening mechanism to prevent lung cancer death. In fact, the US Preventive Services Task Force now recommends Spiral CT scans for all smokers and former heavy smokers between the ages 55 and 79.[5]

The USPSTF cites a lifetime benefit of 5/1,000 lung cancer deaths averted in people who have regular spiral CT screening. But, as stated in the report, screened smokers have 675/1,000 false positive tests, many of which lead to further unnecessary testing. In fact, subjects who had CT scans had 9/1,000 more biopsies or surgeries for benign lesions than did non-screened subjects. The USPSTF does state that it is unclear how beneficial or harmful a screening program will be when instituted in the general population [7].

In 2011 the NLST team published the results of its 5-year study examining the impact spiral CT scans would have on the diagnosis of lung cancer in smokers and ex-smokers. The study involved 53,000 smokers and heavy ex-smokers ages 55–74. Participants were either given a spiral CT or a chest x-ray annually for 3 years, then followed for a total of 5 years. Any positive finding on the CT was followed by subsequent CT scans to assure stability. If the findings were deemed unstable or high risk, patients were put through further diagnostic tests such as PET scans or, if still concerning, lung biopsies. If cancer was detected by biopsy, then typically it was surgically removed. The study reported a significant reduction in lung cancer death among the CT subjects compared to the chest x-ray subjects, as more cancers were identified and cured early in that group [8].

When looking at absolute numbers, 1,060 people in the CT group had cancer diagnosed (almost half of which were diagnosed clinically and not by CT findings), while 941 cancers were discovered in control subjects. The cancer death rate was

---

lower in the CT group (356 vs 443) presumably because more early stage lung cancers were detected and removed. This is a cancer death rate of 13.3/1,000 in the CT group vs 16.6/1,000 in the control group. The survival advantage from lung cancer deaths averted was 3.3/1,000 people screened with CT scans over the 5 years (or 0.66/1,000 screened each year). The overall survival advantage in the CT group (from all causes, not just cancer) was 4.6/1,000 people screened over 5 years. It is unclear why the overall survival advantage may have been higher than the lung cancer survival advantage, since in theory spiral CT scans would only benefit the detection and treatment of lung cancers, and this is something that the authors do not adequately address. It is possible that the people in the non-CT arm were overall a sicker group and thus had a higher death rate.

In the NLST data, spiral CT screening did lead to a large number of false positives. In the CT group, 390/1,000 screened had at least one abnormality detected by CT, and 233/1,000 people without cancer in the CT group had abnormal findings requiring further study typically by PET scan or biopsy. Overall in the CT group 6/1,000 without cancer suffered major complications from interventions.

An earlier study of spiral CT scans in former heavy smokers further illuminates the false positive rate. In this study of 1,035 smokers and former smokers who received a spiral CT scan annually for 2 years, 298 people had abnormal findings (288/1,000 screened). Overall 22 had lung cancer diagnosed (21/1,000), while 95 people needed to have PET scans (92/1,000 screened) and six people had lung biopsies (5.8/1,000) for what proved to be a non-cancerous false positive [9].

Lung biopsies are not without risk. It is estimated that 170–260/1,000 of people develop pneumothorax, 10–140/1,000 need a surgical chest tube placed, and 40–270/1,000 develop pulmonary hemorrhage [10]. In addition, people subjected to annual CT scans are vulnerable to radiation damage. One study estimated that with low-dose spiral CT scans done on 55-year olds, the lifetime excess cancer risk was as high as 1.2/1,000 in women and 0.6/1,000 in men [11]. That risk is likely much higher when people receive PET scans, which is typically performed after a positive spiral CT scan. PET scans deliver almost ten times the radiation of a spiral CT, or the equivalent of 700 x-rays.

A further confounding variable in spiral CT screening is the detection and surgical removal of cancers that would not have been lethal if left alone. Many cancers regress, stabilize, or shrink, and thus cause no harm, yet these cancers would be surgically removed if detected by CT screening. This is significant since in the NLST data 120/1,000 subjects with cancer suffered major complications from surgical removal.

A subsequent look at the NLST data showed that 180/1,000 of all cancers found and removed were indolent and would not have led to death or harm if they had been left alone [12]. That means that 7.1/1,000 people screened, received unnecessary surgery due to the CT findings for cancers that would not have killed them. According to some experts in diagnostic testing, lung surgery is a risky procedure, especially among smokers many of whom have baseline poor health. It is estimated that 50/1,000 people who undergo lung surgery die within 30 days of the operation. Says Gilbert Welch: "Spiral CT technology is detecting a very different category of lung cancer, small abnormalities that meet the pathologic criteria for lung cancer yet are not destined to cause symptoms or death." [13] Time will tell if the NLST survival advantage will persist when CT screening is introduced to the general population, but likely there will be a large number of PET scans and unnecessary biopsies and surgeries performed due to widespread screening, something that will need to be balanced against the mortality improvement derived from early detection of some cancers.

References

1. Villeneuve, P. J., & Mao, Y. (1994). Lifetime probability of developing lung cancer, by smoking status, Canada. *Canadian Journal of Public Health, 85*(6), 385–388.
2. Wao, H., et al. (2013). Survival of patients with non-small cell lung cancer without treatment: A systematic review and meta-analysis. *Systemic Reviews, 2*, 10.
3. Welch, H. G., & Black, W. (2010). Overdiagnosis in Cancer. *Journal of the National Cancer Institute, 102*(9), 605–613.
4. Patz, E. F., et al. (2000). Screening for lung cancer. *The New England Journal of Medicine, 343*(22), 1627–1633.
5. Imhof, H., et al. (2003). Spiral CT and radiation dose. *European Journal of Radiology, 47*(1), 29–37.
6. Storrs, C. (2013). How much do CT scans increase the risk of cancer? *Scientific American, 309*(1).
7. De Koning, H., et al. (2014). Benefits and harms of computed tomography lung cancer screening strategies: A comparative modeling study for the US preventive services task force. *Annals of Internal Medicine, 160*(5), 311–320.
8. NLST Research Team. (2011). Reduced lung-cancer mortality with low-dose CT screening. *New England Journal of Medicine, 365*, 395–409.
9. Pastorino, V., et al. (2003). Early lung cancer detection with spiral CT and positron emission tomography in heavy smokers: 2 year results. *Lancet, 2003*(362), 593–597.
10. Wu, C., et al. (2011). Complications of CT guided percutaneous needle biopsy of the chest. *American Journal of Review, 196*(6), 678–682.
11. Berrington de Gonzalez, A., et al. (2008). Low dose lung CT screening before age 55: Estimates of the mortality reduction required to outweigh the radiation-induced cancer risk. *Journal of Medical Screening, 15*(3), 153–158.
12. Patz, E. F., et al. (2014). Overdiagnosis in low-dose computed tomography screening for lung cancer. *Journal of the American Medical Association Internal Medicine, 174*(2), 269–274.
13. Welch, *Overdiagnosed* (pp. 67–69).

Chapter 10
Health Effects of Smoking

Mr. B had come to a point in his life where he wanted to focus on improving his health. Almost 60 years old, he had newly diagnosed diabetes, and while mild and easily treated, it frightened him. He also had well-controlled hypertension. He worked as an educator in a fairly stressful and busy position. He had very little time to exercise. He was also 50 pounds overweight.

During our visit Mr. B talked about his intent to find time for exercise and to join a weight loss group like weight watchers. We also discussed stress management. But it was I who had to bring up another problem that he did not like to mention.

"What about your smoking?" I asked him. "Don't you think it's time to start working on that?"

As with many of my smokers, Mr. B was well aware of the harm he inflicted upon himself from smoking, but he never liked to bring it up. To him smoking cessation was impossible to achieve. He had tried. And further, as he explained to me, this was not the best time to try again. If he wanted to lose weight, he certainly could not think about quitting smoking, and without cigarettes he did not know how he could contend with his stress. He smoked about a half a pack of cigarettes a day, usually out of sight from his colleagues and his family. Frankly, the fact that he continued to smoke embarrassed him, but quitting scared him more.

We discussed the health risks of smoking, as well as the benefits of quitting. I showed him some hard data, since years of research had clearly delineated the extent of smoking's harm. "I know you want to lose weight," I told him, "but I can't show you any good data that tells me how much your weight loss will impact your health, although I would imagine that it is not in the same stratosphere as what you would achieve from quitting smoking. Especially with diabetes, the risk of heart attack and stroke will be much higher if you continue to smoke than if you quit."

Mr. B struggled during our conversation. I tried to convince him that in fact weight loss, exercise, and smoking cessation could occur simultaneously; in my experience with patients who smoke, those who initiated an exercise program as they quit helped make the latter easier. I also told him about various tools that could help him to quit, from medicines to counseling. He looked again at the numbers.

© Springer International Publishing Switzerland 2015
E. Rifkin, A. Lazris, *Interpreting Health Benefits and Risks*,
DOI 10.1007/978-3-319-11544-3_10

"I guess I'm fooling myself if I keep smoking," he said. "Everything else I can do would seem meaningless unless I quit. Well, I guess now is the time. Let's do it."

Three months later Mr. B was smoke free, had begun to exercise, and lost some weight. Although his weight loss was not as dramatic as he had hoped, he was still satisfied, and actually felt much better. He had a smile on his face and knew that if he could accomplish this, everything else would be easy.

A. Key Questions

- How serious are the health risks that 42.1 million Americans tacitly accept by continuing to smoke?
- Are the data which correlates smoking with lung cancer, oral cancer, coronary heart disease, emphysema, stroke, cervical cancer, reduced fertility, COPD and other chronic debilitating diseases robust?
- Is there any controversy regarding the health risks attributed to smoking?
- If a patient stops smoking, what is the likelihood of reducing disease risk?

B. Risks and Benefits

- We could talk about the risk of contracting any one of the diseases associated with smoking. But some smokers will escape these afflictions, while some non-smokers will contract these diseases. In the end, how will you know whether you got heart disease because you have a family history of heart disease, because you were a lifelong smoker, or both?
- What we can compare are death rates. Everyone dies. But death rates among smokers are discernibly different than those among non-smokers of the same age, so these statistics are a way to quantify the risk of smoking in terms that are easy to understand.
- Even so, absolute information about the health risks associated with smoking can be difficult to interpret. Significant health end points occur after many decades, so we need long-term data on real people as they live their different lives.
- But cigarettes have changed over the last century; so have people's smoking habits, in terms of factors such as how much they smoke and what age they start. Even the people who smoke are different: men used to smoke more than women, but now the proportions are close to being equal.
- And while smoking used to be common throughout American society, it is now most prevalent among the underprivileged: about a third of people below the poverty line smoke, compared to the national average of 21.5 % [1, 3].
- **We can use a Smoking BRCT to illustrate the 198 extra deaths over 25 years associated with 1,000 smokers in the Seven Countries Study when compared**

with **1,000 non-smokers (Fig.** 10.1). **This visual technique dramatically illustrates the health impacts associated with smoking.**

- **Hoping to learn about the long-term effects of smoking cigarettes, other researchers collected information on the lifelong smoking habits of nearly 35,000 male doctors in the UK. The British Doctors Study [6] lasted 50 years, from 1951 through 2001. The researchers observed higher death rates among smokers, in particular due to heart disease, stroke, cancer, and respiratory diseases. Longevity has been increasing rapidly for non-smokers over the past half century, but this was not true for the smokers in the study. Figure** 10.2 **contains a series of BRCTs demonstrating risks from smoking over a 50-year period.**

- Findings from this study show that male cigarette smokers born between 1900 and 1930 died, on average, 10 years younger than men born in the same period who never smoked. Men who quit at age 60, 50, 40, or 30 gained back about 3, 6, 9, or 10 years of life, respectively [6].

- On the whole, lifelong smokers had a lower chance of living into old age. For example, the researchers reported on the survival of men born from 1900 to 1910 who lived from age 35 through age 80 [6]. Nineteen percent of the smokers died in their 40s or 50s compared to 9 % of the non-smokers.

BRCTs:
Health Effects of Smoking

Additional Risks of Death from Many Causes Attributed to Smoking

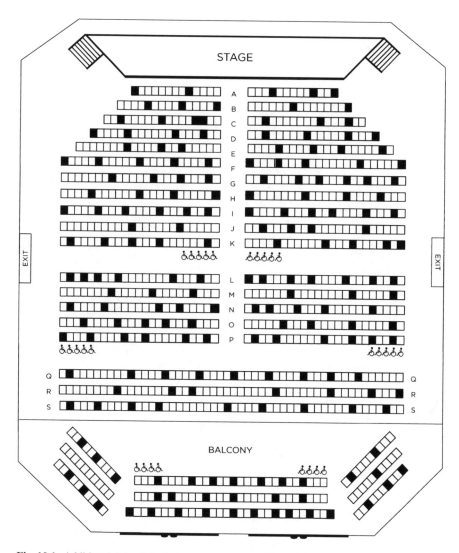

Fig. 10.1 Additional risks of death from many causes attributed to smoking. The Seven Countries Study— the darkened seats in this theater of male smokers represent the 198 extra deaths observed over 25 years compared to a theater of male non-smokers. Of these 198 extra deaths, 52 were from heart disease, 49 were from lung cancer, 40 were from other kinds of cancer, 21 were from chronic obstructive pulmonary disease, and the remaining 36 were from a variety of other causes

The British Doctors Study

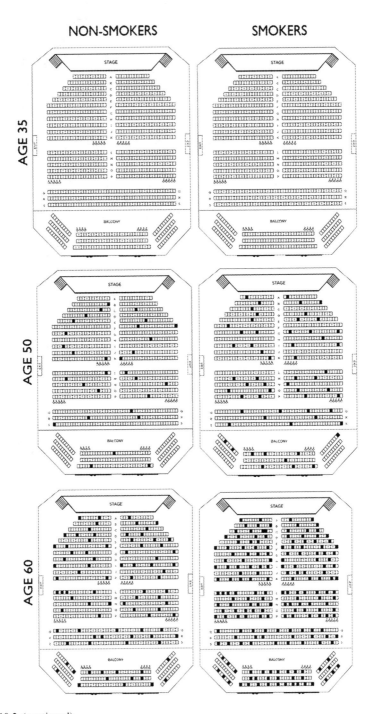

Fig. 10.2 (continued)

NON-SMOKERS   **SMOKERS**

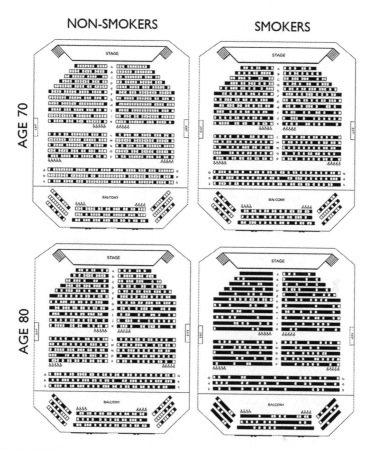

Fig. 10.2 The British Doctors Study—these diagrams represent two groups of 1,000 male British doctors who were born 1910–1919. They were all alive at age 35, as shown in the first, *all-white* BRCTs. The *darkened seats* in each subsequent BRCT show how many of these men died by each age milestone. The BRCTs on the *left* represent non-smokers, while those on the *right* represent smokers

C. Discussion

The subject of smoking has flooded the media since the first reports of adverse health effects appeared 50-some years ago. Public health campaigns, scientific research, the anti-tobacco lobby, and cigarette company trials have all contributed to bring about such a change in the public conscience as would have been unimaginable half a century ago. In 1965, almost half of all American adults were cigarette smokers. By 1985, the proportion of adult smokers had fallen to about 30 % [1]. In the late nineties, California introduced anti-smoking legislation, and many other places followed suit. In 2003, New York City banned smoking in bars and restaurants [2].

According to the CDC, more than 20 % of the US adult population still smokes [3]. An estimated 42.1 million people, aged 18 years or older, in the United States smoke cigarettes [1]. Cigarette smoking is more common among men (20.5 %) than women (15.8 %) [1]. Cigarette smoking is the leading cause of preventable death in the United States; more than 16 million Americans suffer from a disease caused by smoking [2].

In order to make health risk data easier to interpret, researchers do their best to account for complicating factors. Often they use statistical methods. While these studies are far from "perfect," the picture that emerges is still sobering. In 1964, researchers collected information on a large number of middle-aged men living in five European countries, the US, and Japan. Twenty- five years later, they published a follow-up to their Seven Countries Study, confirming "the association of cigarette smoking with elevated risk of mortality from all causes, several cardiovascular diseases, cancer, and chronic obstructive pulmonary disease." [4]

By the end of the study, the participants were hardly youngsters any more. The risk of disease or death may or may not depend on smoking, but it definitely depends on age. So the researchers used statistical methods to attempt to account for the contributions of aging when they analyzed the results. They used similar methods to try to account for a number of other factors as well. This way they could report "standardized" risks, which may be more meaningful especially for comparisons with different studies.

The absolute increase in risk for these smokers was determined to be 198 deaths per thousand over 25 years (Fig. 10.1). The researchers were confident in this result: the statistical probability of observing such an extreme difference between the two groups just by random chance would have been miniscule.

Among the participants smoking 20–29 cigarettes per day, deaths per thousand could be broken down as follows: 168 deaths from coronary heart disease (vs. 116 among non-smokers), 60 from lung cancer (vs. 11 among non-smokers), 28 from chronic obstructive pulmonary disease (vs. 7 among non-smokers), and 111 from other cancers (vs. 71 among non-smokers). Other heart and arterial disease, stroke, infection, accidents, and other diseases accounted for the additional 194 deaths per thousand among the smokers during the 25-year period.

Hoping to learn about the long-term effects of smoking cigarettes, other researchers collected information on the lifelong smoking habits of nearly 35,000 male doctors in the UK. The British Doctors Study [5] lasted 50 years, from 1951 through 2001 (Fig. 10.2). The researchers observed higher death rates among smokers, in particular due to heart disease, stroke, cancer, and respiratory diseases. Longevity has been increasing rapidly for non-smokers over the past half century, but this was not true for the smokers in the study. Male cigarette smokers born between 1900 and 1930 died, on average, 10 years younger than men born in the same period who never smoked. Men who quit at age 60, 50, 40, or 30 gained back about 3, 6, 9, or 10 years in life respectively [5].

On the whole, lifelong smokers had a lower chance of living into old age. For example, the researchers reported the survival of those men born from 1900 to 1910 who lived from age 35 through age 80 [6]. Nineteen percent of the smokers died in their 40s or 50s, compared to 9 % of the non-smokers. The difference in risk became more extreme with age. We have used a series of Smoking BRCTs to provide a rather sobering view of increased risk from smoking cigarettes.

Scientific reports have linked smoking with many different health effects. And as the medical studies continue, the list only grows longer. A single study is rarely "proof" that smoking causes disease X, but the body of research that now exists is extensive enough that scientists and doctors have been able to draw some confident conclusions.

The 2004 US Surgeon General's Report on the Health Consequences of Smoking [6] reviewed and cited over 1,600 different sources. Taken all together, some of this evidence is so convincing that the Report infers a cause and effect relationship between smoking and certain diseases: lung cancer, oral cancer, bladder cancer, cervical cancer, coronary heart disease, stroke, chronic obstructive pulmonary disease (emphysema and chronic bronchitis), reduced female fertility, premature delivery, even cataracts, to name a few.

Other evidence is a bit weaker, merely "suggesting" a causal relationship between smoking and e.g., liver cancer or erectile dysfunction. And according to the Report, we do not know enough to be able to claim that smoking causes decreased sperm quality or adult asthma. In these instances, the authors of this book would classify smoking as risk factor for these conditions.

On the other hand, the Report is satisfied that certain other diseases, like breast cancer, simply are not caused by cigarettes. Smoking even has an occasional health benefit: the Report finds that the evidence is strong for a causal relationship between active smoking and reduced risk of preeclampsia in pregnant women.

Surgeon General's Warning: Smoking Causes Lung Cancer, Heart Disease, Emphysema, And May Complicate Pregnancy – Cigarette Package Warning

If the conclusions of the Surgeon General's Report are not convincing enough, the results of the Seven Countries Study and the British Doctors Study clearly illustrate that smoking cigarettes is detrimental to human health. Regardless of which diseases are associated with smoking and the uncertainty in the exact number of cancers caused by cigarettes, it is clear that smoking significantly increases the risk of death at any age. Nonetheless, we each have the right to decide for ourselves the level of health risk that we find acceptable.

References

1. National Center for Health Statistics (2005). *Health, United States, 2005, with chartbook on trends in the health of Americans.* U.S. Government Printing Office, Hyattsville, Maryland, 535 pp.
2. Perez-Pena, R. (2003). *Smoking ban relies on voluntary compliance.* The New York Times, March 28.
3. Centers for Disease Control and Prevention. (2002). Cigarette smoking among adults – United States, 2002. *Morbidity and Mortality Weekly Report, 53*(20), 427–431.
4. Jacobs, D. R., Adachi, H., Mulder, I., Kromhout, D., Menotti, A., Nissinen, A., & Blackburn, H. (1999). Cigarette smoking and mortality risk: twenty-five-year follow-up of the Seven Countries Study. *Archives of Internal Medicine, 159*, 733–740.
5. Doll, R., Peto, R., Boreham, J., & Sutherland, I. (2006). Mortality in relation to smoking: 50 years' observations on male British doctors. *British Medical Journal, 328*(7455), 1519–1527.
6. U.S. Department of Health and Human Services (2004). *The health consequences of smoking: A report of the Surgeon General.* U.S. Department of Health and Human Services, Centers for Disease Control and Prevention, National Center of Chronic Disease Prevention and Health Promotion, Office on Smoking and Health, Atlanta, GA. Chapters available online at www.cdc.gov.

Chapter 11
Exercise Stress Tests

Mr. S was in his late 50s and had admittedly lived a very sedentary life. He was obese and did not eat well. He did not exercise. He had quit smoking several years earlier but did have a long smoking history. His job was stressful. He had well controlled high blood pressure, and this year he was diagnosed with mild diabetes. Now he decided to make changes in his life.

We talked about dieting, and he had chosen to pursue a fairly vigorous low calorie weight loss regimen, which had started to already strip pounds from his waist. Now he wanted to begin an exercise program. But having done so little, he worried about his risk of exercise without first checking to make sure his heart was in good shape. At his request we performed an EKG, which was unremarkable. Now he inquired about getting a stress test.

Mr. S had no family members with heart disease at a young age, although his father did have bypass surgery in his 70s and his mother died too early to know if she may have had cardiac problems. None of his siblings had known disease, but none were as obese as he, nor did they have diabetes or hypertension. Mr. S traveled often, and he experienced no significant shortness of breath while walking through airports or cities. He never felt chest pain or heart palpitations. If he walked quickly he could be a bit winded, but as soon as he slowed down he felt better.

We talked about the pros and cons of stress tests. Several options for testing existed. He could have a regular treadmill test where he walked on a treadmill and technicians monitored any change in his EKG. He could have the same test with the addition of thallium, a radioactive substance injected into his vein that helped determine if specific areas of the heart were receiving diminished blood flow. He could have an echocardiogram after the administration of a substance called dobutamine, allowing the technician to watch for any decrease in heart wall motion during stress, something indicative of blood flow restriction. Or he could have a CT scan that looked for calcium build-up in his blood vessels that had some correlation with blood vessel blockages. We discussed the pros and cons of these approaches.

"I wonder if you should get any of these tests at all," I suggested. "I'm not sure what we are even going to do with the results."

© Springer International Publishing Switzerland 2015
E. Rifkin, A. Lazris, *Interpreting Health Benefits and Risks*,
DOI 10.1007/978-3-319-11544-3_11

I showed him the known data on stress testing and the fact that there is little information about the benefits of such testing in preventing significant cardiac events, such as heart attacks. Although he did have risk factors for heart disease (obesity, diabetes, high blood pressure, male gender) he had no significant cardiac symptoms of concern. After our discussion he was most concerned about the false-positive rate of stress tests: the fact that so many abnormal tests occurred even in people without heart disease.

"What if that happens?" he asked. "I have to do more tests?"

I told him that the only way to confirm the validity of an abnormal stress test was to conduct more testing, likely an invasive test called a catheterization. I also told him that some people with perfectly normal stress tests have died suddenly from heart attacks. I finally suggested to Mr. S that he had a very low risk of having any heart trouble from exercise, that a stress test likely would not help very much to stratify that risk, and that his health would greatly benefit from exercise and weight loss regardless of whether or not he had heart disease.

In the end, Mr. S chose to eschew the stress test and leaped into a vigorous exercise program. He lost weight. His blood pressure and sugar improved and he felt much better.

A. Key Questions

- Is the patient at high risk of having cardiac disease? This can include a long smoking history, poorly controlled diabetes or hypertension, past or current vascular disease, a strong family history of early heart disease, advanced age, and male gender.
- How often do stress tests help prevent serious cardiac events in asymptomatic people?
- How often do stress tests cause harm in asymptomatic people?
- If the patient does have a positive stress test, how often will those results be false positives? What needs to be done to prove that there is or is not a true heart blockage?
- If the patient does have a normal stress test, how confident can the patient be that he/she will not have serious cardiac disease?
- How well do stress tests predict who will and will not have a cardiac event or cardiac death?
- If a patient is found to have significantly blocked arteries as a result of stress tests, will revascularization with stents or bypass surgery help them?

B. Risks and Benefits

- **It has been determined that approximately 19/1,000 people without cardiac symptoms may benefit from having a stress test by reducing cardiac events and cardiac death (Fig. 11.1).** In these cases the stress test will identify a high-risk blockage that can then be repaired or treated medically, thereby preventing a heart attack.

- **Studies show that about 20/1,000 people without cardiac symptoms will suffer serious harm from having a stress test by increasing unnecessary revascularization procedures that lead to death and stroke. Many more will have serious adverse effects from unnecessary testing and treatment, such as cardiac catheterizations, while still others will be labeled falsely with heart disease based on stress test results (Fig. 11.2).** In these cases a stress test will identify a blockage that, if left alone, would not have caused harm, but in repairing the blockage the patient is medically injured.

- In individuals with abnormal stress tests, 760–978/1,000 people at low risk have no heart disease and 540–930/1,000 people at high risk have no heart disease despite the positive test. The majority of positive stress tests, then, are false positives, and despite the positive test the patient is not at risk for having a cardiac event. Many of these people will have unnecessary invasive and potentially risky cardiac catheterizations to prove that they do not have heart disease. Some of these people will be subjected to unnecessary procedures and medical interventions that can also cause harm.

- It has been found that 3–10/1,000 people with normal stress tests have serious coronary artery disease that is missed by the test. **In addition, most people (650/1,000 men and 470/1,000 women) who present with a heart attack or sudden cardiac death have blockages that would not have been identified by stress testing (Fig. 11.3).** Therefore, a normal stress test does very little to reassure patient or doctor that the patient is not going to have a serious cardiac event.

- As a predictive tool for cardiac events and death, stress tests do not accurately assess who is at high and low risk for poor outcomes. Only 60/1,000 people with abnormal stress tests will have a cardiac events within seven years of the test, while 800/1,000 people who suffer a cardiac event in that time period will have had a normal stress test.

- In people who are found to have significant coronary artery disease by stress testing and subsequent catheterization, approximately 30/1,000 of them will benefit from revascularization (stents, bypass). Others may benefit from medication treatment, although that number is not well documented. Despite this, many low-risk blocked arteries found by stress testing are "fixed" with stents and bypass despite the fact that such procedures have not been shown to improve outcome and can, in fact, cause harm.

BRCTs:
Exercise Stress Tests

Effectiveness of Stress Tests in Preventing Significant Heart Disease in Asymptomatic People

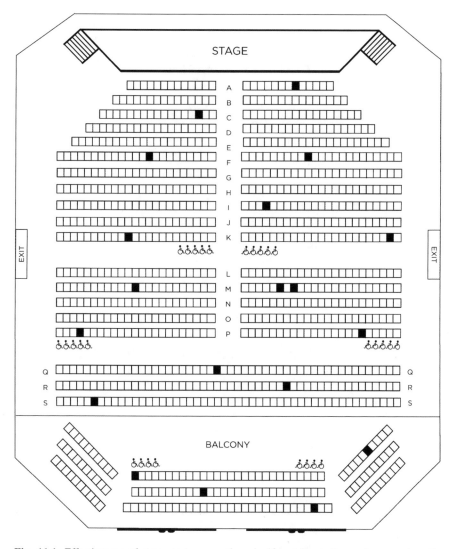

Fig. 11.1 Effectiveness of stress tests preventing significant heart disease in asymptomatic people. Out of 1,000 people in a theater without symptoms who have a screening exercise stress test, approximately 19 of them, represented by the blackened seats, will have a significant cardiac event averted compared to 1,000 people who do not have a stress test

Risks from Stress Testing

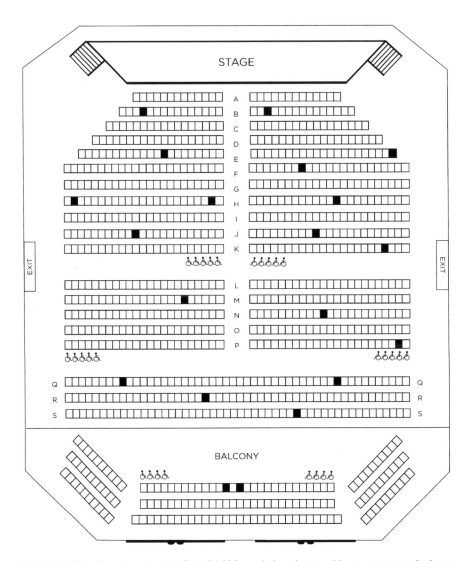

Fig. 11.2 Risks from stress testing. Out of 1,000 people in a theater without symptoms who have a screening exercise stress test, approximately 20 of them, represented by the blackened seats, will suffer substantial harm compared to 1,000 people who are not tested. Such harm usually occurs from additional tests and procedures that are conducted due to either false-positive tests or for lesions found to be clinically insignificant, and could include stroke or heart attack. Overall out of 1,000 abnormal stress tests, 800 are false-positives in people without clinically significant heart disease, and many require potentially dangerous tests to prove that they have no worrisome heart blockages. Some are labeled as having heart disease despite that fact that they are not at risk for cardiac events

Correlation between Normal Stress Test Results and the Absence of Significant Heart Disease

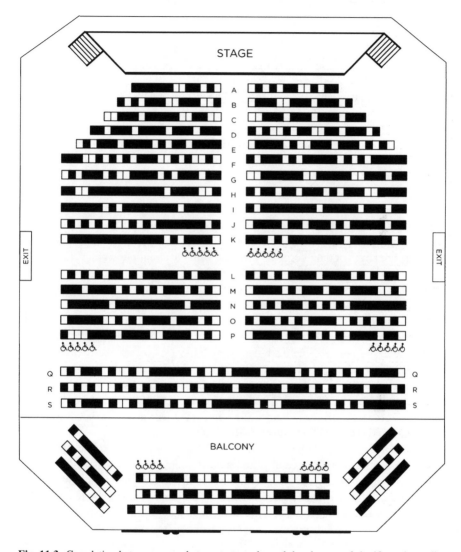

Fig. 11.3 Correlation between normal stress test results and the absence of significant heart disease. Out of 1,000 people in a theater who have a heart attack or who die suddenly from a heart condition, 650 of them, represented by the blackened seats, would have a normal stress test prior to the event. Most cardiac events occur in people with normal coronary arteries that would not be picked up by stress tests

C. Discussion

Coronary artery disease is a specter that hangs over us because of its harsh consequences and its unpredictable nature. It claims many lives and sparks significant
disability, especially as we age. Every year in the United States 715,000 people
suffer heart attacks and 385,000 people die of coronary artery disease. Many people
with vascular heart disease have symptoms such as chest pain, increasing shortness
of breath, and decreased exercise tolerance. Others, though, have as their first
symptom a heart attack or sudden death. In fact, 400/1,000 of all cardiac deaths are
from sudden death, typically in people with no indication of having cardiac problems (see [9]). Certain risk factors can increase the chances of a person having heart
disease, such as diabetes, high blood pressure that is poorly controlled, previous
vascular disease (such as stroke, angina, peripheral vascular disease), obesity, inactivity, and a strong family history.[1]
   It is tempting to seek a means of determining if a patient is at higher risk for
heart disease, both to prevent heart attacks and sudden death, and to institute treatment. Stress testing and CT angiogram are two common non-invasive means of
accomplishing that goal. The objective of either test is to determine which patients
may have blockages of their coronary arteries, with the assumption being that fixing
or treating those blockages will lead to fewer heart deaths. In an ECG stress test,
various changes in the ECG that are triggered by exercise can predict who may have
coronary artery disease and be vulnerable to heart attacks.
   Adding injections of a radioactive substance such as Thallium to the stress test
can theoretically increase the test's sensitivity. Thallium will light up in a patient's
coronary arteries, and those with a blockage will have slower uptake after exercise.
Finally, CT angiograms are a form of CT scan that can identify calcification of coronary arteries, something that is predictive of blockages of those arteries. If any of
these tests are positive, cardiologists will often have to place a catheter into the
arteries to more definitively delineate the coronary artery anatomy and determine
the location and severity of any blockages.
   If a blockage is detected on a stress test or CT angiogram, will that lead to a treatment that can mitigate risk? Actually, finding and fixing most blocked cardiac arteries by means of stents or bypass surgery has not been demonstrated to alter outcome.
Nortin Hadler estimates that of those patients found to have significant (over 50 %)
blockages with screening, only 30/1,000 have blockages (left main disease or proxi-
mal LAD disease primarily) in which aggressive intervention with stents or bypass
surgery lead to better outcomes (fewer deaths and heart attacks) than conservative
medical care. He also notes that when one artery is blocked, typically other arteries
are blocked downstream of that, and thus only a small proportion of a patient's coronary artery disease can be ameliorated through invasive intervention [1, 2].
   Brownlee, in her study of the medical delivery system, shows that as the rate of
stenting has increased in this country, the rate of MI (Myocardial Infarction) has not
declined. While no study has demonstrated the efficacy of using stents in most cases

---

[1] http://www.cdc.gov/heartdisease/facts.htm.

of CAD for blocked arteries, one study showed that only 300/1,000 of stents were deemed medically appropriate by cardiology chart review, while 140/1,000 of stents and 100/1,000 of bypass surgeries were considered absolutely inappropriate [3]. Several large studies, such as the COURAGE trial, have been conducted that verify the conclusions of Hadler and Brownlee that, in most cases, invasive repair of blocked arteries does not lead to meaningful reduction of heart attack and death when compared to simple medical treatment of symptomatic cardiac disease [4–6, 12].

Because stress tests and CT angiograms lead to so many catheterizations, stents, and bypass procedures, and because revascularization has not been shown to alter outcome in most cases, it can be argued that many patients who undergo those screening tests are subjected to subsequent harmful tests and procedures unnecessarily. Cardiac catheterizations can injure femoral arteries, cause severe allergic reactions and serious kidney damage, and even damage the heart vessels they are studying; they do instigate a small number of strokes and heart attacks as well. If patients receive stents based on stress test results these can have similar adverse effects in addition to leading to cardiac vessel rupture, sudden myocardial infarction, and cardiac death.

Bypass surgery is an even more potentially deleterious procedure. According to research done by Brownlee, 10–20/1,000 of patients receiving bypass die from the procedure and 450/1,000 suffer cognitive decline. Several studies have documented a high prevalence of mental status changes caused by bypass [7]. As a surgery, bypass can also induce morbidity in other ways, from prolonged chest wall pain to infection to organ damage. Brownlee estimates that stents cost $3.4 billion a year, and total invasive cardiac procedures could cost as much as $100 billion annually. The personal cost to a patient, though, is more significant, especially if the procedure does not improve clinical outcome and can induce harm. The fact that so many invasive procedures are triggered by findings derived by stress tests, it is important that such tests be ordered rationally and that patients are aware of the ramifications of that testing, both positive and negative.

Several studies have explored the value of resting EKG and exercise stress tests in risk stratifying patients for coronary artery disease. There is little consensus as to their efficacy. The US Preventive Services Task Force recommends against screening with resting or stress EKG tests for low-risk patients without symptoms, and finds that the data is insufficient to recommend for or against testing in patients at high risk. Their review of the literature concludes that no study has demonstrated that stress testing helps better stratify patients into a high or low-risk pool, or that such testing can reduce cardiac death.[2]

An American Heart Association statement in 2005 similarly recommended caution in regard to stress tests [8]. The statement bases its recommendation on available studies and notes that many people who undergo such tests and who do not have predisposing symptoms are given nebulous results. "Indeed, when used as a purely diagnostic test, it must be realized that false-positive tests are common among asymptomatic adults, especially women, and may lead to unnecessary testing, overtreatment, and labeling," the report concludes. The report also notes that

---

[2] http://www.uspreventiveservicestaskforce.org/uspstf/uspsacad.htm.

"randomized trial data on the clinical value of screening exercise testing are absent; that is, it is not known whether a strategy of routine screening exercise testing in selected subjects reduces the risk for premature mortality or major cardiac morbidity." Therefore, even if a positive test does indicate some degree of heart disease, it is unclear if that revelation leads to treatment that improves death rate or quality of life.

The false-positive rate of stress tests can be very high. Multiple studies have demonstrated a wide variance in the accuracy of stress tests. One pooled analysis suggests that in positive stress tests for low-risk patients, only 22–240/1,000 patients will be shown to have disease (false-positive rate of 760–978/1,000), while in high-risk patients the false-positive rate is 540–930/1,000. If thallium is added to the test the false-positive rate can approach 500/1,000 people tested in asymptomatic patients [9] (Also see [10]). In addition, the definition of a "positive" test is not well delineated. Therefore, many people are labeled as having heart disease falsely and even potentially treated for a disease they do not have, and many people are subjected to invasive catheterizations to prove that in fact they do not have heart disease, both of which can be dangerous to the patient.

True positive stress tests identify arteries that have a greater than 50 % blockage, but do not stipulate if those blockages are high risk and would confer benefit if treated. If the goal of stress testing is to identify those people who are likely to die from heart disease or have a major heart attack unless an intervention is provided, then stress tests data is much less reliable and poorly defined [10]. Since many positive stress tests identify low-risk single vessel disease that often does not require treatment, many patients are either catheterized or treated for positive tests without improving outcome and with potentially causing harm.

Stress testing also has significant false-negative findings: People with negative tests who are told they are "normal" may be at high risk of serious heart disease. Popular television journalist Tim Russert is a well-known example of a man who died suddenly of a heart attack soon after having had a normal stress test. It is felt that 3/1,000 people with normal stress tests die of heart attacks within a year of the test [11]. Other studies suggest that between 4 and 10/1,000 people will have cardiac events each year after a normal stress test (see [10]) David Fein of the Princeton Longevity Center estimates that 650/1,000 men and 470/1,000 women have as their first symptom of cardiac disease either a heart attack or sudden death, most of whom would not be identified by stress testing. In fact, a majority of people who present with a significant cardiac event have minor blockages of their arteries, often less than 40 %, something that would not be detected by CT angiogram or even cardiac catheterization. Dr. Fein also notes that adding thallium to the test does not improve the outcome.[3]

Of the people identified as having coronary artery disease by stress testing, has their outcome improved as a result of the test? There have been no definitive studies that determine the value of stress tests in preventing death or serious cardiac

---

[3] http://www.theplc.net/Cardiac_Stress_Tests.html.

outcomes when performed on low risk, asymptomatic patients, or even high-risk patients (see [10]). According to a recent review, it is felt that over 10 years, as many as 19/1,000 symptomatic high-risk patients could benefit from having stress tests that discover high-risk blockages that are repaired by invasive procedures, reducing the rate of heart attack and cardiac death.

The same review also speculates that as many as 20/1,000 symptomatic patients will have an excessive number of strokes, heart attacks, cancer, or death over the same time period as a result of having false-positive stress tests that lead to unnecessary angiograms and invasive procedures [12]. This analysis used a small VA study of very high-risk patients to arrive at the conclusion that up to 27/1,000 of people receiving a stress test will be found to have high-risk lesions whose repair should improve outcome [13]. The analysis does not take into account the possible adverse consequences of performing stents and bypass on patients with true positive stress tests but who have blockages that have not been shown to benefit from such procedures, which constitutes the majority of people found to have coronary artery disease. Therefore, likely more than 20/1,000 patients will suffer harm as a result of their stress test due to the excessive number of invasive procedures performed due to stress test findings showing low-risk blockages.

A study did try to answer the question asked by Mr. S: Will a stress test help determine a patient's risk of exercising? Looking at a large cohort of asymptomatic men with high cholesterol who had stress tests and were followed for over 7 years, the authors attempted to ascertain how good the tests were at predicting cardiac events, such as heart attack or myocardial death. As it turned out, 940/1,000 people with a positive stress test did not have a cardiac event. Contrarily, of those people who did have a cardiac event, 800/1,000 had a negative stress test [14]. Therefore, stress tests did very little to predict who was vulnerable to coronary heart disease and who was not.

References

1. Hadler, The Last Well Person, pp. 27-9.
2. Hadler, *Rethinking aging* (pp. 54–55).
3. Brownlee, *Overtreated* (pp. 101–102).
4. Henderson, R. A., et al. (2003). Seven year outcome in the RITA-2 trial: coronary angioplasty vs. medical therapy. *Journal of the American College of Cardiology, 42*, 1161–1170.
5. Pfisterer, M., et al. (2003). Outcomes of elderly patients with chronic symptomatic coronary artery disease with an invasive vs. optimized medical treatment strategy. *Journal of American Medical Association, 289*(9), 1117–1123.
6. Boden, W. E., et al. (2007). Optimal medical therapy with or without PCI for stable CAD. *New England Journal of Medicine, 2007*(356), 1503–1516.
7. Newman, M. F. (2003). Longitudinal assessment of neurocognitive function after CABG. *New England Journal of Medicine, 344*(6), 395–402.
8. Lauer, M., et al. (2005). Exercise testing in asymptomatic adults: A statement for professionals from the American heart association council on clinical cardiology, subcommittee on exercise, cardiac rehabilitation, and prevention. *Circulation, 112*, 771–776.

9. Vesely, M., & Dilsizian, V. (2008). Nuclear cardiac stress testing in the era of molecular medicine. *Journal of Nuclear Medicine, 49*(3), 399–413.
10. Fowler-Brown, A., et al. (2004). Exercise tolerance testing to screen for coronary heart disease: A systematic review for the technical support for the U.S. preventive services task force. *Annals of Internal Medicine, 140*(7), W9-24.
11. Brody, J., (2008). *The treadmill's place in evaluating hearts.* The New York Times
12. Arbab-Zadeh, A., et al. (2012). Exercise tolerance testing to screen for coronary heart disease: A systematic review for the technical support for the U.S. preventive services task force. *Heart International, 7*(1), e2.
13. Massie, B., et al. (1993). Scintigraphic and ECG evidence of silent CAD in asymptomatic hypertensives. *Journal of the American College of Cardiology, 22*(6), 1595–1606.
14. Sisovick, D. S., et al. (1991). Sensitivity of exercise ECG for acute cardiac events during moderate and strenuous physical activity. *Arch Intern Med, 151*, 32.

Chapter 12
The Use of Warfarin in Atrial Fibrillation

Mr. W was at wit's end. He knew that he had to keep taking this drug, but he was not going to do it silently. "Whose great idea was it to use rat poison to make us better?" he asked me. "The guy should be shot."

Mr. W was inflicted by a condition called atrial fibrillation (afib), an irregular heart rhythm not uncommon in patients of his age. He was now 77 years old. With afib his heart raced rapidly and irregularly, often for no perceivable reason. He took drugs to slow his heart, and now he hardly noticed the problem. But even without symptoms, the mere presence of afib can cause a clot to form in the heart and lead to a higher risk of stroke. The only way to reasonably mitigate that risk is for patients to take a blood thinner like Coumadin™ (Warfarin), which, as Mr. W correctly stated, is also used as a rat poison.

But in some patients Warfarin use can be problematic, and Mr. W seemed to fit in that category. Its dose needs to be kept within a very narrow therapeutic range. Warfarin dose is measured either by means of a blood test or finger-stick, and its results are translated into a number called an INR. If the INR is too low the risk of stroke increases, but if the INR jumps too high, serious bleeding can occur. Many factors can cause wild fluctuations in INR including foods such as salad and other vegetables, vitamins, medicines, and any number of medical conditions.

"So now my number is too high again?" he asked me incredulously, since only two weeks ago his number was low and we decided not to make a medicine adjustment. "I'm not surprised, because my nose is bleeding every morning. I even think I saw blood in the toilet yesterday, although I try not to look. Why does this keep happening?"

We marched through a litany of possibilities. What did he eat? Had he taken any new medicines or vitamins? Did he have a cold? Nothing seemed to be revealing.

"I can't keep living like this," he said. "Part of me just says to heck with it, and I'll just stop taking it and suffer the consequences. It's getting on my nerves. I'm afraid to put anything in my mouth. I'm afraid one day I'll start to pee and a gush of blood will fly out."

© Springer International Publishing Switzerland 2015
E. Rifkin, A. Lazris, *Interpreting Health Benefits and Risks*,
DOI 10.1007/978-3-319-11544-3_12

"We can stop it," I suggested. "You can always take aspirin. That does help too."

"Yea, well my heart doctor says that aspirin is worthless, and that if I stop the Coumadin I'll get a stroke. That's not the way I want to check out, doc. And he won't let me stop it even if I want to. He says there are newer meds that can replace the Coumadin, but they're a lot of money, way more than I can afford, and my insurance won't pay a dime. But he says the newer ones, you don't have to check blood with those, and you can eat whatever you want."

"That's true," I told him, "but they have their problems too. For one thing, if you start bleeding on them you can't stop the bleeding for a few days. At least with Coumadin you can reverse it. And I know that you bleed a lot."

"So then what do I do?" he asked desperately.

I realized that likely no one had talked to him about his risk of stroke on Warfarin compared to if he took aspirin instead. Typically people are prescribed Warfarin the minute they are found to be in afib, and they are never given an opportunity to stop it. Doctors quote a 50 % risk reduction of stroke for those who use Warfarin rather than aspirin. I showed Mr. W the absolute risk reduction of Warfarin compared to aspirin of getting a disabling stroke. I told him that his risk may be a bit higher due to his age and the fact he had high blood pressure. I also showed him the risk of bleeding on Warfarin compared to aspirin.

He seemed very surprised by the charts. "That's not nearly as bad as I thought," he told me. "They said that Coumadin cuts my risk in half. That doesn't look like cutting anything in half. The way I read it, not many people get strokes at all even without the rat poison."

Mr. W told me that he would talk to his wife and think about it. Sometime later he informed me that he decided to stay on the Warfarin and put up with all of its problems, at least for now. Even the slight risk of getting a stroke was too much for him. But if the situation became worse, he told me, he may very well change his mind.

A. Key Questions

- Is there a way to determine the risk of ischemic stroke in a patient with atrial fibrillation, and what is the approximate risk of a disabling stroke?
- Does Warfarin mitigate the risk of a disabling stroke? If so, what is the benefit of using Warfarin over using a drug such as aspirin?
- Are there risks of using Warfarin? Are certain patients at higher risk than others?
- Are there other reasons a patient may benefit from aspirin, such as having had a heart attack, which would make it a better choice than Warfarin? Are there benefits and/or risks of combining Warfarin with aspirin?
- Would the patient be willing and able to contend with the dietary and medication restrictions mandated by the use of Warfarin, would they be compliant with the medicine, and would they reliably obtain the frequent blood work necessary to

monitor INR? Are there other reasons the patient would benefit from taking aspirin, such as a recent heart attack, that would increase the bleeding risk if he/she also took Warfarin?
- Are newer anti-coagulants a better option than Warfarin?

B. Risks and Benefits

- Atrial Fibrillation (afib) does confer an increased risk of ischemic stroke. Most strokes are not disabling, and patients fully recover, but 20–25/1,000 people with afib are vulnerable to clinically significant strokes every year. That risk is higher in people over the age of 70, with poorly controlled hypertension and diabetes, with congestive heart failure, and with a past history of stroke.
- **The use of blood thinners like Warfarin does reduce the risk of clinically significant ischemic strokes. Compared to patients who take aspirin or other anti-platelet agents, people on Warfarin have 6–10/1,000 fewer disabling ischemic strokes in a year. Patients with more risk factors have a higher likelihood of having a stroke on aspirin compared to Warfarin (Fig. 12.1).**
- The primary risk of Warfarin is the development of serious bleeds. The rate of serious bleeds per year among patients on Warfarin is 38/1,000; for the elderly the rate is 70/1,000. Further, 17.4/1,000 additional people on Warfarin visit hospitals for major bleeds, and 3.2/1,000 die from their bleeds compared to those not taking Warfarin.
- **When compared to those on aspirin, patients with afib on Warfarin have an additional 12/1,000 major bleeds and 6/1,000 hemorrhagic strokes (Fig. 12.2).**
- Some patients take aspirin or other anti-platelet agents for other medical reasons, such as coronary artery disease. If Warfarin is added to those medicines, there is no additional risk reduction in ischemic stroke, but there are 90/1,000 additional bleeds in a year when compared to people on Warfarin alone.

BRCTs:
The Use of Warfarin in Atrial Fibrillation

Effectiveness of Warfarin in Preventing Stroke in People with Afib

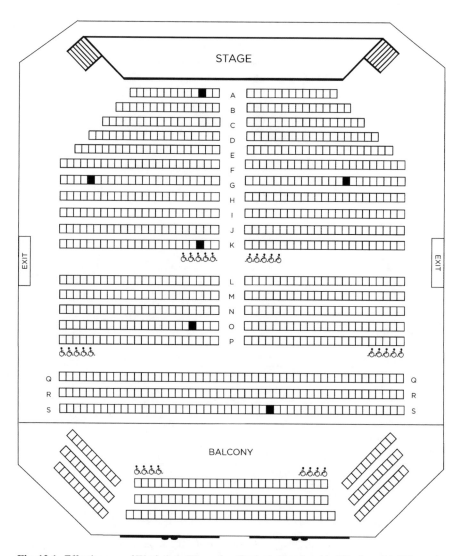

Fig. 12.1 Effectiveness of Warfarin in Preventing Stroke in People with Afib. Out of 1,000 people with atrial fibrillation sitting in a theater and deemed to be at moderate risk of stroke who take Warfarin, approximately 6, represented by blackened seats, disabling strokes will be prevented in a year compared to 1,000 people who take aspirin

Risks Associated with Taking Warfarin

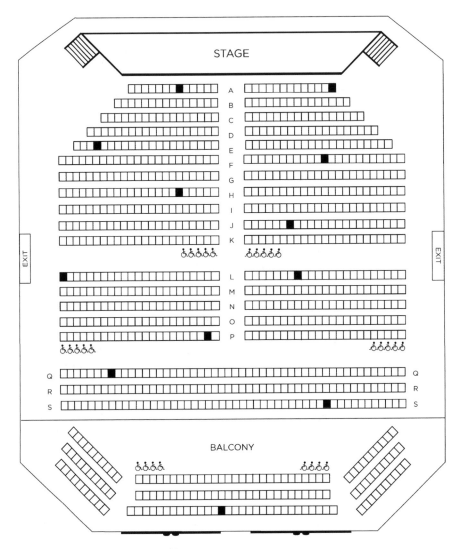

Fig. 12.2 Risks Associated with Taking Warfarin. Out of 1,000 people with atrial fibrillation sitting in a theater and deemed to be at moderate risk of stroke who take Warfarin, approximately 12, represented by blackened seats, more of them will suffer major bleeds compared to 1,000 people who take aspirin. This includes an excess of 6 people out of 1,000 who bleed in their brains compared to 1,000 people who take aspirin

C. Discussion

Atrial Fibrillation (afib) is an irregular heart rate that becomes more common as people age. Any condition that stretches or strains the atria—sustained high blood pressure, congestive heart failure, valvular heart disease, lung disease, heart surgery, or even age itself—can instigate afib. Typically, especially in older patients, once the rhythm begins it is very difficult to extinguish. Patients can present with heart palpitations, dizziness, chest pain, and shortness of breath. Some who have weaker hearts can be pushed into congestive heart failure. With medication, most of the symptoms of afib can be controlled, and the risk of cardiac complications is similarly mitigated.[1]

The primary risk of afib, especially when its symptoms are controlled, is that of ischemic stroke. The atria do not contract well in afib, and thus a clot can build up on its walls. If that clot becomes dislodged, it can travel through the blood stream and block blood vessels leading to the brain, causing a stroke. About 2.7 million Americans have afib, although many do not know that they have the condition. Stroke, which is the fourth highest killer in the country, is five time more common in afib patients than in the regular population, and it is thought that 150/1,000 of all stokes can be ascribed to afib.[2] By anti-coagulating the blood, either with anti-platelet agents such as aspirin or with anti-coagulants such as Warfarin, it is less likely for afib patients to develop a clot, and thus less of a chance for them to have an ischemic stroke.

Without a doubt, Warfarin decreases the risk of ischemic stroke in patients with afib, even when compared with aspirin. Since stroke can be so devastating, it is now considered standard of care to treat most afib patients with Warfarin, especially if they have one of the high-risk conditions defined by the CHADs score. These include age over 70, high blood pressure, congestive heart failure, diabetes, or a past history of stroke or mini-stroke [1]. Without any CHAD risks, then it is felt that aspirin is adequate to prevent strokes in afib patients. But especially in the elderly, when the CHAD score and subsequently the risk of stroke are deemed to be too high to justify the use of aspirin, Warfarin is given without pause.

Multiple studies corroborate the CHAD score's prognostic power, and several calculators exist whereby patients can determine their stroke risk with afib. For example, a 75-year-old person without other risk factors may have a 28/1,000 risk of having a stroke. If that patient also has high blood pressure, the risk rises to 40/1,000.[3] There is very little data about the size and extent of the strokes that people in afib studies suffer, and even whether or not they are at all disabling, since many strokes are silent and lead to no persistent symptoms. Also, there is still uncertainty about

---

[1] http://my.clevelandclinic.org/heart/atrial_fibrillation/afib.aspx.

[2] http://www.strokeassociation.org/STROKEORG/LifeAfterStroke/HealthyLivingAfterStroke/UnderstandingRiskyConditions/When-the-Beat-is-Off---Atrial-Fibrillation_UCM_310782_Article.jsp#.

[3] http://www.qxmd.com/calculate-online/cardiology/chads2-stroke-risk-in-atrial-fibrillation.

how accurate and clinically applicable scales like CHAD are to any particular patient [2, 3]. Overall since approximately 700/1,000 people with strokes make a full recovery (see chapter on carotid screening), it is important to know what the risk reduction of permanently disabling strokes is for both Warfarin and aspirin in patients with afib, and what the possible adverse effects are of those two therapies.

Most studies suggest a 50 % annual risk reduction (using relative risks) of ischemic stroke in afib patients who take Warfarin vs. aspirin, a number that varies marginally based on the CHAD score. But what is the absolute risk reduction of disabling stroke? In several studies the aggregate risk of stroke is approximately 25/1,000 annually in patient with afib, and that risk can be cut in half with Warfarin to less than 10/1,000 [4]. But those numbers, while significant, are not as dramatic as they appear for two reasons. First, the overall stroke risk is decreased also by use of aspirin, although not as much as Warfarin, so it is best to compare Warfarin to aspirin. Second, since less than half of strokes cause permanent disability, most people with afib who develop stroke will make a full recovery.

By some studies, people deemed to be at risk for stroke (higher CHAD score) have a 40–50/1,000 risk of having an ischemic stroke in a year without treatment. With aspirin that risk is 25–38/1,000 and with Warfarin the risk is 14–18/1000. Assuming that half of the strokes will be non-disabling, the use of Warfarin in high-risk patients with afib prevents 6–10/1,000 disabling strokes in a year compared to those who use aspirin[4] [5]. It is important to note that the risk of stroke is not cumulative over years; for instance, if the risk of stroke is 6/1,000 in one year, that does not imply that over 5 years the risk will be 30/1,000.

Warfarin does have its risks that need to be considered when assessing its utility. Some of the risks, which were apparent in the case of Mr. W, are difficult to measure. These involve the very fickle nature of Warfarin and the need to regularly monitor it. Warfarin is a medicine cursed by having a narrow therapeutic window; when too low it is ineffective, and when too high it causes bleeding. Warfarin levels are measured either by a finger-stick or standard blood test, and results are reported in a range called the INR. Typically patients with afib are expected to maintain an INR between approximately 2 and 3. But levels can vary widely, and many medicines, foods, and illnesses can dramatically alter a patient's INR.

Some patients have a very difficult time controlling their levels even when they adhere to a strict diet and maintain a stable medicine regimen. Others find the dietary restrictions to be too difficult to follow. Still others are on a fluid number of medicines and supplements that can potentially send INR levels in many directions on any given day. The need to fall within Warfarin's narrow window can impact a patient's lifestyle and even impart harm in those patients subject to fluctuations and, although such an effect cannot be quantified and put in a BRCT, it may certainly influence decision-making, as it did with Mr. W.

The primary complication of Warfarin is its risk of causing bleeds. While bleeding is more likely when the INR increases beyond the upper limit of normal, bleeds can occur even within the therapeutic window. Several studies have attempted to

---

[4] http://www.aafp.org/afp/2005/0615/p2348.html.

measure the rate of bleeds in patients who take Warfarin. Some have found the bleeding rates higher than others and many have found more bleeding in patients who are older or who have higher CHAD scores.

Bleeds can be minor, such as a bloody nose, or can be major, such as a gastrointestinal hemorrhage or even a bleed in the brain, which is called a hemorrhagic stroke. In a recent study of patients with afib on Warfarin, 38/1,000 patients suffered a major hemorrhage in a year, 17.4/1,000 visited the hospital for a major bleed, and 3.2/1,000 people died as a result of their bleed. In another study of only older patients, the rate of serious bleeds was 70/1,000, some of which were fatal [6, 7]. When compared to aspirin treated patients with afib, those treated with Warfarin had 12/1,000 more major bleeds in a year, and 6/1,000 more intracranial bleeds, which is another form of stroke [8].

Also, patients who are on anti-platelet drugs such as aspirin or Clopidogrel™ have even a higher risk of bleeding without any additional reduction in stroke risk when they simultaneously take Warfarin. One study showed an increase yearly bleed risk of 92/1,000 in patients on Clopidogrel™ and Warfarin compared to those on Warfarin alone [9]. Certainly patients who have a high propensity for bleeds (ulcers, nose bleeds, colon lesions), and who have unsteady balance and are prone to falls, may have even more likelihood to have serious bleeds on Warfarin. In fact, Warfarin itself may lead to more falls and fractures according to another study, so like with many drugs, each patient has to assess his or her own risk profile before deciding whether the medicine is appropriate [10].

There are newer medicines with similar efficacy as Warfarin in preventing stroke in afib without having the same number of interactions or as narrow a therapeutic window, such as Dabigatran™ and Apixaban™ [11]. In fact, these new drugs do not require any medicine/dietary restrictions and do not necessitate blood monitoring. But they have one tremendous side effect: they cause similar rates of bleeding as does Warfarin, and it is far more difficult to stop bleeding with the newer medicines. If a patient develops a significant hemorrhage on Warfarin he/she can be given vitamin K and the anti-coagulation effect will quickly reverse the situation. If a patient develops a significant hemorrhage on one of the newer drugs, the effect of the drug could persist for days, making the bleed even more dangerous. In addition, the newer drugs are very expensive, and they have other side effects that are becoming more prevalent the longer the medicines are on the market. In our opinion, while we looked only at Warfarin, the newer drugs will have similar BRCTs but with unique additional issues.

References

1. Gage, B. F., et al. (2001). Validation of clinical classification schemes for predicting stroke: results from the national registry of atrial fibrillation. *Journal of American Medical Association, 285*(22), 2864–2870.
2. Hart, R., & Pearce, L. (2009). Current status of stroke risk stratification in patient with atrial fibrillation. *Stroke, 2009*(40), 2607–2610.

3. Fang, M. C., et al. (2008). Comparison of risk stratification schemes to predict thromboembolism in people with nonvalvular atrial fibrillation. *Journal of the American College of Cardiology, 51*(8), 810–815.
4. Go, A. S., et al. (2003). Anticoagulation therapy for stroke prevention in atrial fibrillation: how well do randomized trials translate into clinical practice. *Journal of American Medical Association, 290*(20), 285–292.
5. Mant, J., et al. (2007). Warfarin versus aspirin for stroke prevention in an elderly community population with atrial fibrillation: The Birmingham atrial fibrillation treatment of the aged study, BAFTA: A randomized controlled trial. *Lancet, 370*(9586), 493–503.
6. Gomes, T., et al. (2013). Rates of hemorrhage during warfarin therapy for atrial fibrillation. *Canadian Medical Association Journal, 2013*(185), E121–E127.
7. Fihn, S. D., et al. (1996). The risk for and severity of bleeding complications in elderly patients treated with warfarin. *Annals of Internal Medicine, 124*(11), 970–979.
8. The Stroke Prevention in Atrial Fibrillation Investigators. (1996). Bleeding during antithrombotic therapy in patients with atrial fibrillation. *Archives of Internal Medicine, 156*(4), 409–416.
9. Hansen, M. L., et al. (2010). Risk of bleeding with single, dual, or triple therapy with warfarin, aspirin, and clopidogrel in patients with atrial fibrillation. *Archives of Internal Medicine, 170*(16), 1433–1441.
10. Gage, B. F., et al. (2006). Risk of osteoporotic fracture in elderly patients taking warfarin. *Archives of Internal Medicine, 166*, 241.
11. Connolly, S., et al. (2009). Dabigatan versus warfarin in patients with atrial fibrillation. *New England Journal of Medicine, 361*(12), 1139–1151.

Chapter 13
Aspirin for Prevention of Heart Disease and Stroke

Mrs. L and I looked over her list of medicines, as we did every year during our Wellness visit. I asked her about her over the counter drugs, and she listed a few vitamins and supplements.

"What about aspirin?" I asked.

"Of course," she said. She had not included that in her list.

I asked her why she was taking aspirin, a question that seemed to catch her off guard. She told me that everyone of her age takes aspirin. She was in her lower 60's without many medical problems. She did have high blood pressure well controlled on a single medicine. Her parents both died fairly recently, neither of whom had serious heart disease. She did not smoke and was reasonably active.

She took a single baby aspirin a day, 81 mg. That dose had been recommended in a health letter she read, and most of her friends took the same dose. She never had any difficulties on the aspirin, no bleeding or bruising, no stomach pain. Like with many of her supplements that she ingested, she was taking aspirin just to keep on top of her health. Specifically she did not want to get a heart attack or stroke.

While she took only two prescription medicines she religiously took five supplements daily in addition to the aspirin. These included fish oil and Vitamin E, also to help her prevent a heart attack. She has some mild arthritis and so took Advil™ on occasion, no more than a couple a day. She also had a glass of wine every night.

I talked briefly with her about her individual risk of having a stroke or heart attack. Using a BRCT, we discussed whether aspirin might mitigate that risk. In fact, aspirin might confer a small benefit for her, especially in regard to non-lethal strokes, but her risk was otherwise so low as to make this benefit even smaller. I also showed her data on her other vitamins, explaining to her that several of her over the counter medicines, including the aspirin, could adversely impact kidney function and potentially cause bleeding problems and even ulcers. I did acknowledge that the risks of such worrisome side effects were rare.

© Springer International Publishing Switzerland 2015
E. Rifkin, A. Lazris, *Interpreting Health Benefits and Risks*,
DOI 10.1007/978-3-319-11544-3_13

"But from what you are saying," she said, "I'm not getting anything really useful from taking these things either. Those numbers don't look very impressive. Why does everyone tell us to take an aspirin then?"

I told her that in people with known heart disease or a history of strokes aspirin does convey some benefit, and that people extrapolate such data to assume that everyone should take aspirin. People at high risk for vascular disease also may benefit more than she. In the end, she left my office deciding not to take the aspirin as well as several of her other supplements. But she remained uneasy.

"I felt better thinking that I could take this stuff and prevent something bad from happening. Now I have to actually work at it and go to the gym. Thanks a lot doctor!"

A. Key Questions

- If a patient has had a heart attack or stroke, is he/she at a high risk of developing another cardiac or cerebral event, and will the use of aspirin modify that risk? This is known as secondary prevention.
- If a patient has not had a prior heart attack or stroke, will aspirin improve their likelihood of avoiding these events and living longer? This is known as primary prevention.
- Are there differences in the effects of aspirin between those patients with more risk factors for cardiovascular disease and those with fewer?
- Are there differences in the effects of aspirin between men and women?
- What dose of aspirin is optimal, and how often? At what age should it be started?
- What are the risks of taking aspirin? Are those risks impacted by other medical conditions or other drugs/supplements?
- Are other drugs better than aspirin for primary and secondary prevention?

B. Risks and Benefits

- Aspirin is recommended for secondary prevention. Studies show a 37/1,000 reduction of heart attack vs. placebo, and a 26/1,000 reduction in stroke.
- **For primary prevention in low-risk patients, studies show a 6/1,000 reduction in heart attack vs. placebo. In high-risk patients, there is a 31/1,000 reduction in heart attack (Fig. 13.1).**
- There are differences between men and women. Aspirin is more helpful to prevent heart attacks in men and strokes in women. For primary prevention, men have 6/1,000 fewer heart attacks compared to placebo, but 2.8/1,000 more strokes. Women have no change in heart attacks, and 2/1,000 fewer strokes.

- **The rate of serious bleeding with aspirin in secondary prevention and in primary prevention of high-risk patients is 25/1,000 higher than placebo. For low-risk primary prevention, the excess major bleeds are 4/1,000 people. There were many more minor side effects with aspirin over placebo as well (Fig. 13.2).**
- There is no consensus about the dose and timing of aspirin.
- Several supplements interact with aspirin, including Vitamin E and Fish Oil.
- Other anti-platelet agents such as Clopidogrel™ seem to confer no additional risk reduction compared to aspirin.

BRCTs:
Aspirin for Prevention of Heart Disease and Stroke

Benefits for Healthy People Taking Aspirin

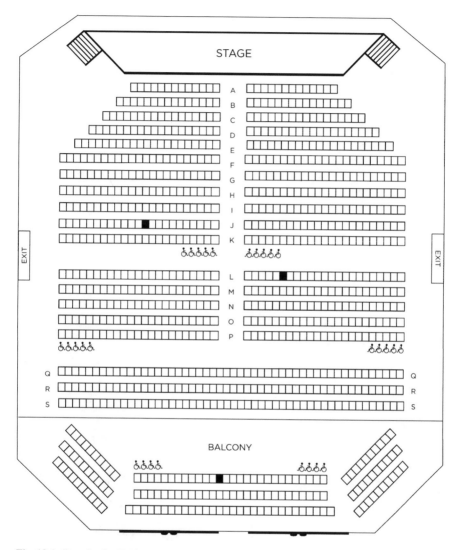

Fig. 13.1 Benefits for Healthy People Taking Aspirin. Of 1,000 healthy men in a theater who take aspirin regularly, approximately 6 will have some reduction in adverse cardiac outcomes compared to 1,000 men who take a placebo, but 3 will have an increase in stroke, so approximately 3 men, represented by blackened seats, will benefit in aggregate. In 1,000 healthy women on aspirin, 2 will have a reduction in stroke risk, but none will have a decrease in cardiac outcomes compared to 1,000 women who take placebo

Risks from Taking Aspirin

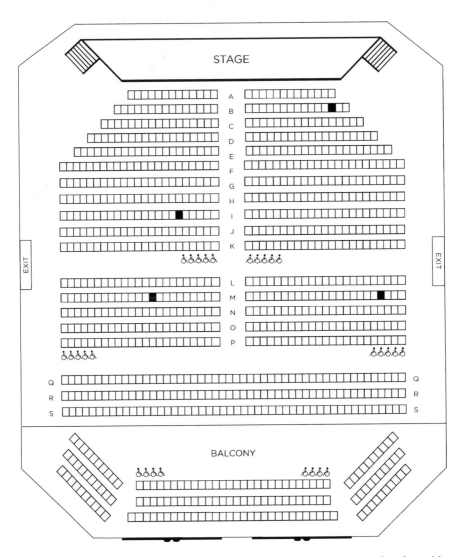

Fig. 13.2 Risks from Taking Aspirin. Out of 1,000 healthy people in a theater who take aspirin regularly, 4 of them, represented by blackened seats, will have a serious gastrointestinal bleed compared to 1,000 people who take placebo

C. Discussion

Aspirin is a well-established anti-inflammatory agent that impedes the action of platelets. While aspirin can cause people to bleed more and heal slower, it can also thwart the platelet-mediated thrombosis that instigates many vascular events. It has historically been used in patients who have acute ischemic (non-bleeding) strokes and heart attacks, often being the first medicine patients receive when they enter the hospital doors. It has also been shown to be helpful to prevent subsequent heart attacks and strokes in patients who have already suffered from a stroke or heart attack and is considered standard treatment for such patients. Such treatment is labeled as secondary prevention, since its goal is to curb the reoccurrence of an adverse event rather than to stop the initial event itself. The latter scenario is called primary prevention and the use of aspirin in that setting is less clear.

Because heart disease and stroke are both devastating and prevalent, and because aspirin seems to be an innocuous intervention that could reduce that risk, many patients and physicians assume that an aspirin a day makes good sense. This is particularly true in patients at high risk of vascular events, such as those who smoke, who have diabetes, who have a positive family history of stroke or heart attack, who have had a previous vascular event, who are sedentary or obese, and in women who use birth control. The risk of bleeding with aspirin varies based on a patient's own individual health status, co-existing medical problems, and prior history. Certain medicines can augment that risk, including two of Mrs. L's supplements: Vitamin E and fish oil.

Currently, the US Preventive Services Task Force recommends the use of aspirin in men between 45 and 79 years old who are at a high risk of having heart disease (including those who have had a prior MI or stroke) and in women between 55 and 79 years old who are at high risk of having strokes. In any patient who is outside that age range, there is insufficient evidence to argue for or against aspirin use in primary prevention. The USPSTF does not delineate the precise risk factors that would sufficiently justify the benefit of aspirin use in primary prevention, nor does it state the dose and timing of aspirin administration that is needed to achieve risk reduction.

According to the USPSTF site regarding pooled studies of primary prevention: "Men in these studies experienced fewer myocardial infarctions, and women experienced fewer ischemic strokes. Aspirin does not seem to affect CVD mortality or all-cause mortality in either men or women. Aspirin use for the primary prevention of CVD events likely provides more benefits than harm to men at increased risk for myocardial infarction and women at increased risk for ischemic stroke."

The USPSTF does stipulate that any patient in whom the risk of serious bleed exceeds the potential benefit should not take aspirin.[1]

Several studies have examined the benefit of aspirin in both primary and secondary prevention of heart disease. A 2009 meta-analysis of six large trials with a total of 95,000 patients over multiple years studied the use of aspirin in both primary and secondary prevention. The dose of aspirin in these studies ranged from 75 to 300 mg a day [1]. The primary prevention group was divided into both high-risk and low-risk subsets. In 2012 the American College of Chest Physicians devised clinical guidelines based on this study [2].

For the primary prevention of low-risk people, there were six fewer MI's per 1,000 treated in the aspirin group and four more major bleeds. In the prevention of high-risk people, there were 31 fewer MI's per 1,000 treated in the aspirin group and 22 more major bleeds. In both high- and low-risk subjects, total death and strokes were unable to be ascertained.

For secondary prevention, there were 37 fewer MI's per 1,000 treated in the aspirin group, 26 fewer strokes, and 25 more major bleeds. There were 13 fewer deaths in the treated group, but that finding was of borderline statistical significance. The study also compared aspirin to Clopidogrel™, a newer anti-platelet agent, in secondary prevention. There was no statistical difference between the two groups.

Several studies look at the unique effect of aspirin on men and women. As noted, the USPSTF recommends the use of aspirin in men who are at high risk of having heart attacks and in women who are at high risk of having strokes, implying that aspirin impacts each sex differently. A 2006 meta-analysis studied the difference in aspirin's effect on men and women in primary prevention [3]. Men did have a reduction of 6.4 heart attacks per 1,000 treated, while women had no change in the MI rate. Women did have a reduction of 2 ischemic strokes per 1,000 treated, while men actually had an increase stroke rate of 2.8. Both groups had an increase in major bleeds, 2.6 per 1,000 treated in women and 3.65 in men. While the overall death rate was slightly lower in women who took aspirin compared to placebo (1.4/1,000), it was somewhat higher in men (3.65/1,000).

A 2005 randomized trial looked specifically at the impact of aspirin on the primary prevention of cardiovascular disease in women [4]. In this trial, 40,000 women over the age of 45 were given aspirin (100 mg) or placebo every other day and monitored for 10 years. Out of 1,000 treated women, there were 2.5 fewer strokes, 1.8 fewer deaths, 0.3 fewer stroke deaths, 0.25 more heart attacks, 8 increased gastrointestinal bleeds, and 6.5 more peptic ulcers than placebo-treated women. This seems to correspond to the generalized finding that aspirin improves stroke risk but not cardiac risk in women. The lower death rate in the aspirin-treated group did not correspond to a lower vascular death rate and has no discernible explanation.

---

[1] http://www.uspreventiveservicestaskforce.org/uspstf/uspsasmi.htm.

References

1. Baigent, C., et al. (2009). Antithrombotic Trialists' (ATT) collaboration aspirin in the primary and secondary prevention of vascular disease: collaborative meta-analysis of individual participant data from randomised trials. *Lancet, 373*(9678), 1849–1860.
2. Per Olav Vandvik, MD Chest. (2012).141(2 Suppl): e637S–e668S. *Primary and secondary prevention of cardiovascular disease antithrombotic therapy and prevention of thrombosis.* 9th ed: American College of Chest Physicians Evidence-Based Clinical Practice Guidelines
3. Berger, J., et al. (2006). Aspirin for the primary prevention of cardiovascular events in women and men: A sex-specific meta-analysis of randomized controlled trials. *Journal of American Medical Association, 295*(3), 306–313.
4. Ridker, P. M., et al. (2005). A randomized trial of low-dose aspirin in the primary prevention of cardiovascular disease in women. *New England Journal of Medicine, 352*(13), 1293–1304.

Chapter 14
Screening for Carotid Disease in Asymptomatic Patients

Mrs. M inquired about several tests she thought she should have. One of them was an ultrasound of her carotid arteries. She had a friend who had a similar test last year, as part of her exam by a very thorough cardiologist, and they discovered a 90 % blockage of one of her arteries.

"If they hadn't done that test," she informed me, "She would have had a stroke. The doctor told her that it was found just in the nick of time; one more month may have been devastating."

I asked my patient a few questions: had she ever had signs of a stroke, i.e., numbness or weakness of one side of the body, slurred speech, a sudden loss of vision in one eye? She had none of these. She was a healthy 75-year-old woman without significant medical problems. She took statin cholesterol medicines, something she carried with her from her prior doctor. Her blood pressure hovered in the high normal range, and she did take a small dose of a blood pressure medicine. Otherwise she was in excellent health without complaints.

"Did your friend get surgery?" I asked her.

"Yes, right away," she said. "It was an easy surgery, she did well, and now she's ok. She said it wasn't even a big deal."

I talked to her about the risks and benefits of getting a carotid ultrasound. If positive, I told her, there was a fair chance that it could be a false positive, and we may have to conduct a catheter test to ascertain the extent of her blockage, a test that itself has a small chance of inducing a stroke. If she did have surgery, that too could cause a stroke. If she did have a tight blockage of her carotid artery found by the ultrasound, some studies suggested that perhaps 25/1,000 such patients would avoid a clinically significant stroke with a surgery. On the other hand, 30/1,000 people who undergo these surgeries have serious complications, including strokes. I showed her the data.

© Springer International Publishing Switzerland 2015
E. Rifkin, A. Lazris, *Interpreting Health Benefits and Risks*,
DOI 10.1007/978-3-319-11544-3_14

"I'm most afraid of the false positives," she told me. "I suppose I can get the test and then see what happens. But then what? How do I know that I won't get a stroke from trying to prevent a stroke?"

I told her to think about it some more; there was certainly no rush. But she had already made up her mind. She decided to forgo the test.

A. Key Questions

- Is my patient at high risk of stroke? What is the likelihood of carotid artery stenosis?
- Do carotid ultrasound tests accurately predict which asymptomatic patients have significant carotid artery stenosis?
- Are there potential harms from carotid artery ultrasounds performed on patients without symptoms of stroke?
- For those asymptomatic people discovered to have carotid stenosis with ultrasound, will they have reduced risk of stroke if they have surgery to open the blockages? Is there any risk of harm from such surgery?

B. Risks and Benefits

- Strokes cause a significant amount of death and disability, although a majority of people with stroke do make a full recovery. It is estimated that 150/1,000 strokes are due to carotid artery disease, with blockages of 60–99 % considered high risk. Many people with carotid blockages have no symptoms until they have a stroke.
- **While carotid ultrasounds can detect high grade blockages in patients without symptoms, they have a high false positive rate. It has been determined that 400/1,000 abnormal carotid ultrasounds occur in patients without significant blockages (Fig.** 14.1**).** People with false positive ultrasounds are not at risk of stroke, but often are subjected to unnecessary testing, and some tests, such as angiograms, confer significant potential risk, including a 10/1,000 risk of causing a stroke.
- There is also a sizable false negative rate, as up to 100/1,000 people with high grade blockages would have a normal ultrasound. Therefore, a normal carotid ultrasound will not rule out the possibility of having a significant carotid blockage.
- People found to have significant carotid blockages by ultrasound screening often undergo carotid surgery. **Carotid surgery in asymptomatic patients over 5 years can prevent 27 disabling strokes out of 1,000 people found to have significant blockages. It is felt that 9,000 people need to be screened with ultrasound to prevent 1 disabling stroke, while causing other harm due to the high false positive rate (Fig.** 14.2**).** That other harm is due to unnecessary angiograms and even surgery.
- **Out of 1,000 asymptomatic people found to have significant lesions by carotid ultrasound who then undergo surgical repair, approximately 30 of them will suffer from a stroke or die during surgery (Fig.** 14.3**).**

BRCTs:
Screening for Carotid Disease in Asymptomatic Patients

False Positives from Carotid Artery Ultrasound Screening

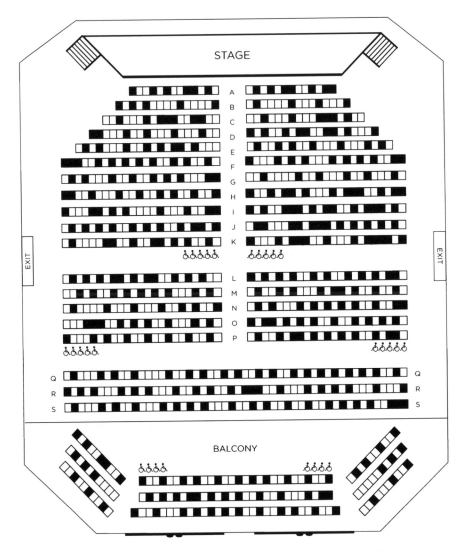

Fig. 14.1 False Positives from Carotid Artery Ultrasound Screening. Out of 1,000 asymptomatic people sitting in a theater who have carotid artery ultrasound screening and are found to have an abnormality, 400 of them, represented by blackened seats, will actually not be found to have any significant carotid disease after further tests are performed. That is a false positive rate of 400 out of 1,000

Stroke Avoidance with Surgical Treatment in Asymptomatic People who have Carotid Lesions Discovered by Screening

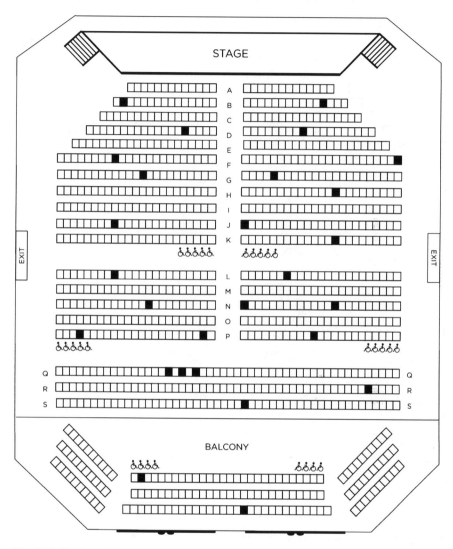

Fig. 14.2 Stroke Avoidance with Surgical Treatment in Asymptomatic People who have Carotid Lesions Discovered by Screening. Out of 1,000 asymptomatic people sitting in a theater found to have significant lesions by carotid ultrasound who then undergo surgical repair, 27 of them, represented by blackened seats, will avoid a disabling stroke within 5 years

Asymptomatic People who have Carotid Lesions
Harmed by Surgical Treatment

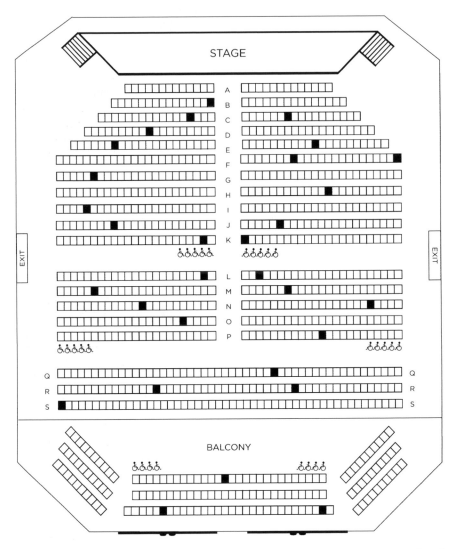

Fig. 14.3 Asymptomatic People who have Carotid Lesions Harmed by Surgical Treatment. Out of 1,000 asymptomatic people sitting in a theater found to have significant lesions by carotid ultrasound who then undergo surgical repair, approximately 30 of them, represented by blackened seats, will suffer from a perioperative stroke or will die during surgery

C. Discussion

Strokes constitute a significant cause of both mortality and morbidity in this country. There are 795,000 Americans who suffer from a stroke every year, and 130,000 die. While strokes can be devastating, and are often felt to be the primary cause of disability in this country, approximately 700/1,000 people with strokes make a full recovery.[1] Most strokes are ischemic, due to either a direct blood clot within one of the brain's arteries, or a clot that travels to the brain's circulation from another site.[2] Many risk factors contribute to stroke, including high blood pressure, smoking, and previous stroke or transient ischemic attack. Some strokes too are caused by blockages of carotid arteries, which are the large blood vessels that supply the anterior of the brain. These vessels can become blocked, or can develop enough plaque that some of it breaks off and obstructs arteries further into the brain. These blockages are called carotid artery stenoses (CAS). It is felt that blockages of 60–99 % constitute some degree of risk.

According to US Preventive Services Task Force data, approximately 1 % of the population has a carotid stenosis greater than 60 %. This number increases with age. Out of all strokes, approximately 150/1,000 of them are due to carotid artery disease.[3] It is tempting to think that finding and repairing blocked carotid arteries may help reduce the overall mortality and morbidity of strokes in patients without any symptoms of stroke. Ultrasounds are the primary tool doctors utilize to ascertain if carotid arteries are blocked. These tests are innocuous, with no direct harmful ramifications. If significant blockages are discovered, patients often will have angiograms to ascertain the extent of the blockages, and can then have carotid artery surgery called carotid endarterectomy (CEA), by which arteries are cleared of plaque. Such surgeries have become more common and less harmful over time.

The US Preventive Services Task Force recommends **against** screening for carotid stenoses with ultrasound in asymptomatic patients. Citing the very low prevalence of CAS in the population, a generalized screening program would lead to a large number of false positives. Several studies have looked at the accuracy of ultrasound detection of clinically significant carotid blockages, and it is generally felt that the tests have a false positive rate of 400/1,000 and a false negative rate of 100/1,000 [1–3]. Based on these studies, 400/1,000 people with abnormal carotid ultrasound in fact have no significant CAS, and 100/1,000 people with normal carotid ultrasounds actually have a significant CAS. Those deemed to have abnormal tests would likely proceed to a more invasive test called an angiogram to ascertain the presence and extent of the blockage. According to USPSTF data, approximately 10/1,000 patients undergoing an angiogram suffer a stroke. Therefore, many people with false positive ultrasounds will have unnecessary testing and be vulnerable to harm without any potential benefit. Also, a sizable number of people with normal

---

[1] http://www.stroke.org/site/DocServer/SSDI_Brochure_FINAL_web.pdf?docID=8281.

[2] http://www.cdc.gov/stroke/facts.htm.

[3] http://www.uspreventiveservicestaskforce.org/uspstf07/cas/casarticle.htm.

ultrasounds actually will have significant carotid disease, but they will be falsely reassured by the false negative test.

A further question is whether even those patients with true positive tests—those proven to have high grade blockages by angiogram—will benefit from CEA. USPSTF pooled data shows that the overall reduction of disabling stroke from carotid surgery in asymptomatic patients with high grade CAS over 5 years is 27/1,000, with more men benefiting than women. CEA itself has its risks. In asymptomatic patients the surgery confers a risk of stroke or death within 30 days of surgery in at least 30/1,000, with higher numbers in smokers and patients with coronary artery disease and hypertension. CEA can also increase the risk of heart attacks near the time of surgery, with a heart attack incidence of 6–33/1,000 within 30 days of CEA.

Overall the USPSTF estimates that 9,000 asymptomatic people would have to be screened and treated over 5 years to prevent 1 disabling stroke, and many people would be over-tested and over-treated due to that screening, leading to significant direct harm. Another pooled analysis suggests that screening men over the age of 65 increases overall quality adjusted life expectancy by an average of 5 days [4].

Two large trials of asymptomatic carotid screening programs comprise the bulk of current data. The ACAS (Asymptomatic Carotid Atherosclerosis Study) trial was published in 1995, [5] and the ACST (Asymptomatic Carotid Surgery Trial) in 2004 [6]. Both trials look at asymptomatic patients with high grade (over 70 %) CAS and compare medical treatment with CEA. The ACAS trial followed people for 2.7 years and extrapolated results to 5 years. They found an advantage of 27/1,000 fewer deaths and major strokes among those receiving CEA. Of note, the cardiac death rate was higher in the non-CEA arm (24 vs. 15), indicating that the non-CEA group may have more underlying severe cardiac disease, which may have falsely exaggerated its overall death rate. In the ACST trial, 3,000 patients were followed for 3.4 years, and the reduction of major stroke or death in the CEA arm was 25/1,000. There was a 31/1,000 perioperative death/stroke rate among those who received the CEA.

References

1. Jahromi, A. S., et al. (2005). Sensitivity and specificity of color duplex ultrasound measurement in the estimation of internal carotid artery stenosis: a systematic review and meta-analysis. *Journal of Vascular Surgery, 41*, 962–72.
2. New, G., et al. (2001). Validity of duplex ultrasound as a diagnostic modality for internal carotid artery disease. *Cathterization and Cardovascular Interventions, 52*(1), 9–15.
3. Adnan, I., et al. (2001). Role of conventional angiography in the evaluation of patients with carotid artery stenosis demonstrated by doppler ultrasound in general practice. *Stroke, 2001*(32), 2287–91.
4. Lee, T. T., et al. (1997). Cost-effectiveness of screening for carotid stenosis in asymptomatic persons. *Annals of Internal Medicine, 126*, 337–46.

5. (1995). Endarterectomy for asymptomatic carotid artery stenosis. Executive Committee for the Asymptomatic Carotid Atherosclerosis Study. *Journal of American Medical Association 273*, 1421–1428

6. Halliday, A., et al. (2004). Asymptomatic Carotid Surgery Trial (ACST) Collaborative Group. Prevention of disabling and fatal strokes by successful carotid endarterectomy in patients without recent neurological symptoms: Randomised controlled trial. *Lancet, 363*, 1491–502.

Chapter 15
Cholesterol Screening

At age 70, Mrs. L was in fairly good health. She remained very active without limitation. She had well controlled high blood pressure, but few other medical problems. Still, she was concerned about her health, especially since so many of her friends and relatives were coming down with illness. Today she came in for a general checkup.

In the past, Mrs. L had been diagnosed with high cholesterol. She even spent some time on various medicines, including statins, which she could not tolerate, and Zetia™, which she stopped due to cost. Both medicines did bring her cholesterol down but she had not checked cholesterol for a few years, and she knew that today was judgment day: She came in fasting so I could check her labs and likely put her on a cholesterol pill. "Why are you worried about your cholesterol?" I asked her.

"Because it's high," she said. "And I don't want to get a heart attack any time soon."

She had looked on the internet and read an article in the health section of the paper that frightened her. It seemed, she said, that a lot of people were getting heart attacks because they were not addressing their high cholesterol. She even handed me a copy of guidelines that suggested that doctors were being too lax in reducing their patients' cholesterol levels.

"I am willing to try something natural, or really work on my diet, or even take the Zetia™ if I have to. I just don't want to go on the statins again," she said. She even stated that she had been eating Cheerios every morning in the hope of getting the cholesterol down for today's test.

We talked about the predictive value of high cholesterol in determining her risk of getting a heart attack. We discussed a recent study showing that among a large number of people who presented with heart attacks, as many of them had low cholesterol as had high. I showed her data about cholesterol and heart attacks. I also talked to her about medicines like Zetia™ and moderate changes in diet.

"Zetia™ and Cheerios can make the number look better," I told her. "But I can't tell you that either, or anything natural, will cut down your risk of heart attack or stroke, or help you to live longer. We just don't have any data to support that."

© Springer International Publishing Switzerland 2015
E. Rifkin, A. Lazris, *Interpreting Health Benefits and Risks*,
DOI 10.1007/978-3-319-11544-3_15

The conversation confused her; she assumed that it was established dogma that people with high cholesterol get more heart attacks, and that by reducing that number the risk of heart attack will diminish. Now, looking at the numbers I showed her, she was less convinced. "Why so much emphasis on the cholesterol, then?" she asked. "Why does everyone always talk about it?"

Given her lack of other risk factors, and her general good health, I could not tell her that checking and fixing her cholesterol would benefit her. I left the decision to her.

"You know what," she said. "Let's skip it. I don't need that kind of stress. If it's not going to help me to know, what's the point? I'm just sorry I had to starve myself today!"

A. Key Questions

- Within a population, do individuals with essentially normal blood serum cholesterol have a lower incidence of coronary heart disease than individuals with elevated levels of blood serum cholesterol?
- Does lowering cholesterol result in a marked reduction in the incidence of coronary heart disease (CHD)? Who determines what constitutes a marked reduction?
- In light of statements from prominent physicians knowledgeable about cholesterol and heart disease, should we worry about elevated cholesterol levels? Who makes the final decision?
- How can we determine if we should be screened for blood serum cholesterol levels, eat cholesterol free food, and take drugs to lower our cholesterol levels? Is this kind of decision based on our level of acceptable risk?
- What is meant when scientists and doctors say that elevated cholesterol is a surrogate for an increased incidence of heart disease?
- Why do we only hear about reduced cholesterol numbers and not reduced deaths from heart attacks when taking cholesterol lowering drugs?

B. Benefits and Risks

- It is assumed that if blood serum cholesterol is lowered, CHD and associated deaths will also be lowered. We now know there is very little empirical evidence to support that view. As is always the case, great care needs to be taken to ask the "right" questions.
- The benefits of cholesterol screening should be based on the reduction of CHD and deaths from lowering cholesterol blood serum levels. Unfortunately, the goal has become lowering cholesterol and, as a result, lowering cholesterol has become a surrogate (e.g., substitute or stand-in) for lowering CHD and associated deaths.

- The only values which are *readily available* are based on how effective drugs (e.g., statins) and dieting are for lowering cholesterol. It's very difficult to find useful information on how lowering cholesterol will reduce CHD and/or associated deaths. Available evidence suggests there is no meaningful correlation.
- **Published clinical studies shed light on the subject and provide the data needed to evaluate absolute risks associated with different blood serum cholesterol levels. Two large clinical studies, which are the most often cited, have shown that essentially the same number of individuals with normal and elevated cholesterol have atherosclerosis and CHD (Fig. 15.1).**
- By definition, cholesterol can be designated a primary risk factor for CHD only if individuals with elevated blood serum cholesterol levels have an appreciably higher incidence of atherosclerosis and CHD than individuals with normal cholesterol levels.
- If 1,000 people had their cholesterol measured before and after taking a statin, there is a high likelihood that almost all of them would have lower blood serum cholesterol values. *However, the significant question would be; does lowering blood serum cholesterol significantly reduce death from CHD. Two very different endpoints!*

BRCT:
Cholesterol Screening

Benefits of Reducing Blood Serum Cholesterol Levels

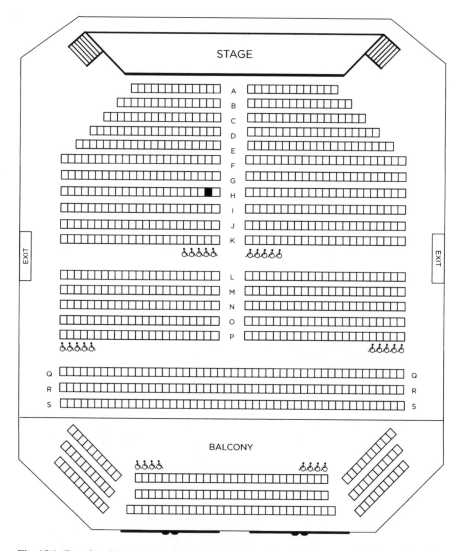

Fig. 15.1 Benefits of Reducing Blood Serum Cholesterol Levels. Represents 1,000 people whose mean total blood serum cholesterol level is 280 mg—a level uniformly characterized as significantly elevated. The darkened seat represents one additional death from CHD when compared to 1,000 individuals with essentially normal cholesterol levels (between 210 and 220 mg)

C. Discussion

Overall, about 600,000 people die of heart disease in the US every year —that is 1 in every 4 deaths [1]. Coronary heart disease (CHD), the most common type, kills nearly 380,000 people in the US annually. Further, over 70 million Americans have some form of cardiovascular disease, which accounted for nearly 40 % of all deaths in the United States at the turn of the twenty-first century [1]. These are frightening statistics. So, it is not surprising that CHD has been attracting intense interest in the public health community for decades. With "baby boomers" aging and more individuals being affected by CHD, this interest will continue to grow. It is increasingly important that we understand CHD so we are more able to reduce or eliminate those factors responsible for this disease.

The prevailing view is that elevated blood serum cholesterol is a primary controllable risk factor (as opposed to uncontrollable risk factors, such as age and genetics) in the development of atherosclerosis and CHD. Reports in the media state rather convincingly that the risk of CHD is markedly lower when blood serum cholesterol levels are lowered; the current benchmark falls in the vicinity of 200 mg/100 ml or less—frequently abbreviated to "200 mg" in everyday speech (please note that this chapter adopts the abbreviated notation). It is also assumed that lowering cholesterol dramatically reduces the risk of suffering and death from atherosclerosis and CHD. This perspective appears to be logical. Since cholesterol is one of the substances that tends to accumulate in arteries and impede blood flow, resulting in atherosclerosis and eventually CHD, lowering blood serum cholesterol levels should reduce the incidence of CHD and death.

It has been estimated that 200 million Americans had cholesterol screening tests, 13 million are on cholesterol-lowering drugs, and 52 million are on cholesterol-lowering diets. In 2001, the Third Report of the National Cholesterol Education Program, a government-sponsored panel, suggested that the number of Americans taking cholesterol-lowering drugs be raised to approximately 36 million, and that more Americans—about 65 million—should be on cholesterol-lowering diets [2]. In 2013, new guidelines laid out in the report *2013 ACC/AHA Guideline on the Treatment of Blood Cholesterol to Reduce Atherosclerotic Cardiovascular Risk in Adults* were issued by the American Heart Association and the American College of Cardiology. Implementation of these new treatment guidelines could raise the number of Americans taking drugs to lower cholesterol to over 70,000,000 [3].

But, as it turns out, the relationship between cholesterol levels and the incidence of CHD is not as clear as popular reports suggest. A doctor at the Harvard Medical School notes that "half of all myocardial infarctions [heart attacks] and strokes occur in individuals without elevated cholesterol levels ...." [4] Cardiovascular pioneer Dr. Michael DeBakey found that elevated cholesterol levels had no effect on the recurrence of coronary disease [5]. Many doctors have spoken of the difficulty with tying heart disease diagnosis to cholesterol levels alone. Dr. William Kannel, one of the first directors of the famous clinical Framingham Study on the relationship of cholesterol levels to CHD, stated that "diagnosis of overt heart disease on the basis of lipid [cholesterol] levels alone is simply not feasible." [6] Dr. William Castelli, another former director of the Framingham study, wrote, "Obviously, the total cholesterol value cannot accurately predict which patients have a [...] problem when the cholesterol levels are between 200 and 250 mg or even between 150 and 250 mg." [7] He also reported that "one-half of all heart attacks now occur in people whose serum cholesterol level is 225 mg or less." Since the average cholesterol level among adult Americans is about 220 mg, his statement means that heart attacks occur almost equally among people with normal and elevated blood cholesterol levels.

Dr. Mark Hegsted, former director of the US Department of Agriculture Human Nutrition Center, observed that the report of the World Health Organization and many others have emphasized how the majority of heart attacks apparently occur in individuals with serum cholesterol levels below 240 mg [8]. In fact, many experts in this field have determined that people with low and high cholesterol have the same number of plaques in their arteries.

So we have a conundrum. We have to look to major, robust, well-respected studies to see if individuals with low blood serum cholesterol levels have fewer deaths from CHD than individuals with elevated cholesterol. The two most frequently cited large clinical studies (e.g., Multiple Risk Factor Intervention Trial (MRFIT) and the Framingham study [9–11]) have shown that nearly the same number of individuals with normal and elevated cholesterol have atherosclerosis and CHD.

Patients might also wonder why these data seem to fly in the face of reports from physicians, drug companies, and government agencies. Why would medical practitioners, agencies like the FDA, and pharmaceutical companies misrepresent the truth? But the answer is not that they are pulling the wool over patient's eyes. It is just that they are presenting results that relate to *nationwide health risks not a patient's individual risks*. They also have their own interests and motives and tend to characterize data in a way that supports their own particular views and perspectives—a trait that we all seem to possess in one form or another.

For example, drug companies almost always use relative numbers to explain the benefits of drugs to reduce cholesterol. As mentioned earlier, this is a valid statistical approach but it makes the benefits from these drugs seem dramatic and, as a result, significantly distorts the risks associated with elevated cholesterol. In addition, government agencies focus on health benefits to the entire nation rather than to the individual.

So hypothetically, if there are approximately 50 million Americans with elevated cholesterol, and if CHD risks for those people are 0.1 % higher than for individuals with normal cholesterol, then 50,000 lives might be saved annually by lowering those people's cholesterol levels.

Bottom line, patients would then have to ask whether an *individual* annual risk of 1 in 1,000 (0.1 %) constitutes an acceptable risk? Is a 0.1 % risk reduction worth modifying diet, changing major lifestyle elements, and taking expensive, potentially dangerous drugs (see Chap. 16 on Statins, Cholesterol and Coronary Heart Disease) in an attempt to lower cholesterol to essentially normal levels or below? Patients would need to decide about levels of acceptable risk and what course of action to take.

Some people may conclude that a 1/1,000 (0.1 %) risk is not worth taking; these individuals may be concerned enough to take action to reduce blood serum cholesterol levels. But others may question whether the increase in the level of risk associated with elevated cholesterol is serious enough to warrant concern.

Another way to look at these results would be to say that for 999 out of 1,000 individuals each year, it makes no difference whether they have elevated cholesterol or normal cholesterol in terms of whether they develop CHD. What are the odds that any patient would be that 1 person? Patients' values, principles, tenets, and concerns about risks and benefits should determine what constitutes an individual acceptable risk.

References

1. Murphy, S. L., Xu, J. Q., & Kochanek, K. D. (2013). Deaths: Final data for 2010. *National Vital Statistics Report, 61*(4), 1–117.
2. Expert Panel on Detection, Evaluation, and Treatment of High Blood Cholesterol in Adults. (2001). Executive summary of the third report of the National Cholesterol Education Program (NCEP) expert panel on detection, evaluation, and treatment of high blood cholesterol in adults (Adults Treatment Panel III). *Journal of American Medical Association, 285*(19), 2486–2497.
3. CarStone, N. J., Robinson, J., Lichtenstein, A. H., Bairey Merz, C. N., Lloyd-Jones, D. M., Blum, C. B., McBride, P., Eckel, R. H., Schwartz, J. S., Goldberg, A. C., Shero, S. T., Gordon, D., Smith, S. C., Jr., Levy, D., Watson, K., & Wilson, P. W. (2013). ACC/AHA guideline on the treatment of blood cholesterol to reduce atherosclerotic cardiovascular risk in adults: A report of the American College of Cardiology/American Heart Association Task Force on Practice Guidelines. *Journal of the American College of Cardiology, 63*(25 Pt B), 2889–2934.
4. Ridker, P. M. (2003). High-sensitivity C-reactive protein and cardiovascular risk: Rationale for screening and primary prevention. *American Journal of Cardiology, 92*(4 supp 2), 17K–22K.
5. DeBakey, M. E., & Glaeser, D. H. (2000). Patterns of atherosclerosis: effects of risk factors on recurrence and survival – analysis of 11,890 cases with more than 25-year follow-up. *American Journal of Cardiology, 85*(9), 1045–1053.
6. Kannel, W. B., Dawber, T. R., Friedman, G. D., Glennon, W. E., & McNamara, P. M. (1964). Risk factors in coronary heart disease: An evaluation of several serum lipids as predictors of coronary heart disease; The Framingham Study. *Annals of Internal Medicine, 61*, 888–899.
7. Castelli, W. P., & Anderson, K. (1986). A population at risk: Prevalence of high cholesterol levels in hypersensitive patients in the Framingham Study. *American Journal of Medicine, 80*(2 suppl), 23–32.
8. World Health Organization (WHO) (1982). *Prevention of coronary heart disease, report of a WHO expert committee.* Technical Report Series No. 678, WHO, Geneva, 53 pp.
9. Kannel, W. B., Castelli, W. P., & Gordon, T. (1979). Cholesterol in the prediction of atherosclerotic disease: New perspectives based on the Framingham Study. *Annals of Internal Medicine, 90*(1), 85–91.
10. Kannel, W. B., Neaton, J. D., Wentworth, D., Thomas, H. E., Stamler, J., Hulley, S. B., & Kjelsberg, M. O. (1986). Overall and coronary heart disease mortality rates in relation to major risk factors in 325,348 men screened for the MRFIT (Multiple Risk Factor Intervention Trial). *American Heart Journal, 112*(4), 825–836.
11. Stamler, J., Wentworth, D., & Neaton, J. D. (1986). Is the relationship between serum cholesterol and risk of premature death from coronary heart disease continuous and graded? Findings 356,222 primary screenees of the Multiple Risk Factor Intervention Trial (MRFIT). *Journal of American Medical Association, 256*(2), 2823–2828.

Chapter 16
Statins, Cholesterol, and Coronary Heart Disease

Mr. C, an 87-year-old man on many medications, came in with his daughter for an initial visit. He lived alone having recently moved to a retirement community to be near his family. He had no significant acute health issues causing alarm. He had been told that he had a heart attack at some point in the past, although he never recalled it nor did his daughter. He had high blood pressure, diabetes, arthritis, poor balance, some increased forgetfulness, and some general aches and pains.

Upon review of his medicines, we found some that he likely did not need, including various vitamins and even some pills for his bowels and bladder that he was convinced never helped him. He was on three blood pressure medicines, although his pressure was very low. He admitted that he felt tired and dizzy at times. He was also on a high dose of a statin (a category of drugs used to reduce cholesterol levels) called Simvastatin.

"Why are you on that?" I asked him.

"High cholesterol," both he and his daughter told me very matter-of-factly. He had been on that medicine for more than a decade.

We talked about stopping some of his blood pressure pills and a few others, but I also questioned whether he needed to be on a statin. Both he and his daughter seemed uncomfortable about stopping it.

"My cholesterol was pretty high before I started it and it's much better now," Mr. C told me. "Plus my heart doctor said I could never go off of it."

Mr. C was unsure why he had been seeing a cardiologist, having no active heart issues, but he was quite adamant that stopping the statin would portend disaster. I talked to him about some potential side effects of his high dose statin, including perhaps some of the muscle pain he experienced. I also showed him how much statins decreased the risk of death and heart attack. Because we did not really know if he had had a heart attack, and because he did have several cardiac risk factors, I showed him how a statin may impact him both if he had heart disease and if he did not.

His daughter peered most intently at the information. "Doesn't seem all that impressive, Dad," she said to Mr. C. "Especially if it's making your legs hurt."

© Springer International Publishing Switzerland 2015
E. Rifkin, A. Lazris, *Interpreting Health Benefits and Risks*,
DOI 10.1007/978-3-319-11544-3_16

We talked a bit more, and agreed to a trial off of the statin to see if indeed any of his symptoms improved without the drug in his body. "How long will it take for me to feel better off it?" Mr. C asked me. "And how long can I be off it before I drop dead?"

I explained that any positive effect of the statin would diminish over many years, so a few months trial off it would cause him no harm. I also suggested that we could always use a lower dose or different statin if he felt the need to stay on it. Walking out with many fewer medicines than when he came in, Mr. C felt a bit apprehensive, but overall very satisfied.

A. Key Questions

- Do individuals taking statins have a lower incidence of CHD when compared to individuals not taking these drugs?
- If so, are the benefits due to lowering blood serum cholesterol levels, or are they due to something else?
- Are the benefits of statins greater for individuals with previous CHD?
- What are the risks of taking statins to the liver, kidneys, muscles, and eyes?
- Is it appropriate to compare the absolute risks and benefits of taking statins in order to make a decision regarding these drugs?

B. Risks and Benefits

- **In primary prevention studies (individuals without previous CHD), an average of approximately 30 out of 1,000 people benefited from taking statins when compared to individuals not taking these drugs. In other words, the average absolute benefit for using statins for primary prevention is about 3 % (3 out of 100). This means that the other 97 % of people taking statins for primary prevention did not benefit from taking these drugs, at least in terms of CHD (Fig. 16.1).**
- **In secondary prevention studies (individuals with previous CHD), an average of approximately 67 out of 1,000 people benefited from taking statins when compared with individuals not taking these drugs. In other words, the average absolute benefit for using statins for secondary prevention is about 7 % (7 out of 100). This means that the other 93 % of people taking statins for secondary prevention did not benefit from taking these drugs, at least in terms of CHD. Therefore, people who have already had a heart attack benefit significantly more from statins than people with no history of CHD (Fig. 16.2).**

- **Statins can cause side-effects and complications like: rhabdomyolysis (muscle destruction); abnormal changes in liver function; kidney failure; myopathy (muscle disease); adverse changes in memory, thinking, and concentration; cataracts; depression and irritability; increased pain, tingling, and numbness; sleep problems; sexual dysfunction; blood sugar changes; and nausea. Side effects can affect a significant number of people (Figs. 16.3 and 16.4).**
- Statins may also play a role in reducing inflammation and blood clots which may lead to reduced prevalence of CHD. Statins can affect the innermost layer of cells lining our arteries (the endothelium), make smooth muscle cells less active, and affect the physiology of the artery wall.

BRCTs:
Statins, Cholesterol, and Coronary Heart Disease

Benefits from Statin Use in Individuals who <u>Never</u> had a Heart Attack (Primary Prevention)

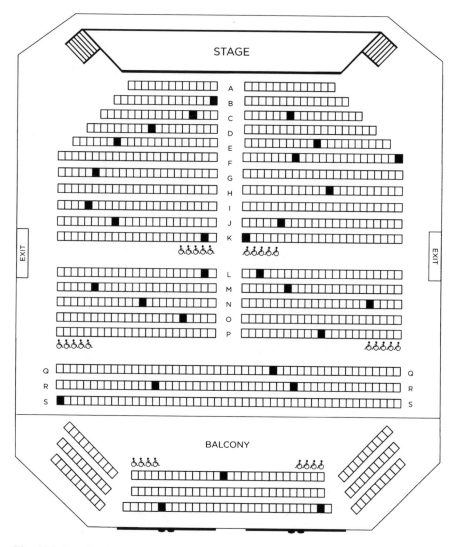

Fig. 16.1 Benefits from Statin Use in Individuals who Never had a Heart Attack (Primary Prevention). Participants in these studies did not have previous cardiovascular disease. The darkened seats (30) represent the average number of individuals out of 1,000 who avoided CHD over a 5-year period by taking statins, as compared to people who did not take statins

Benefits from Statin Use in Individuals who had a Previous Heart Attack (Secondary Prevention)

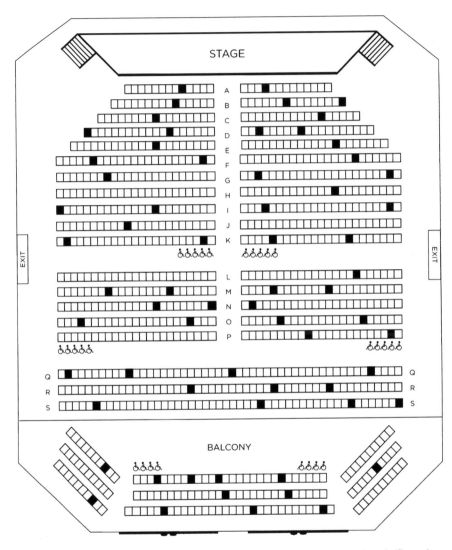

Fig. 16.2 Benefits from Statin Use in Individuals who had a Previous Heart Attack (Secondary Prevention). Participants in these studies had previous cardiovascular disease. The darkened seats (67) represent the number of individuals out of 1,000 who avoided CHD over a 5-year period by taking statins, as compared to people who did not take statins

Cataracts from Statin Use

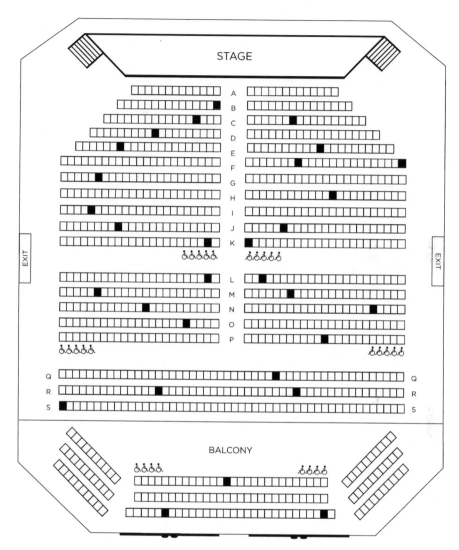

Fig. 16.3 Cataracts from Statin Use. Additional risks from taking statins, represented as darkened seats, include 30 extra patients with cataracts out of 1,000 when compared to 1,000 patients not taking statins

Liver Dysfunction from Statin Use

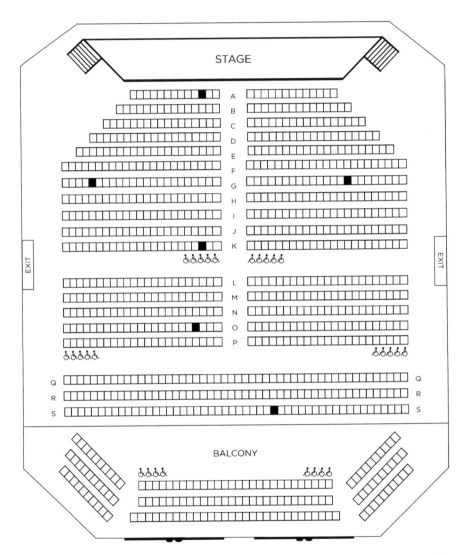

Fig. 16.4 Liver Dysfunction from Statin Use. Additional risks from taking statins, represented by darkened seats, include approximately six additional patients out of 1,000 experiencing liver dysfunction when compared to 1,000 patients not taking statins

C. Discussion

Statins—Vytorin™, Lipitor™, Lovastatin (Mevacor™),Crestor™, Pravastatin (Pravachol™), and Simvastatin (Zocor™) —are the most widely used prescription drugs in the world. More than 214 million monthly prescriptions were written in 2012 [1]. Why are they so popular? People take statins to lower their cholesterol. Indeed, these drugs can reduce blood serum cholesterol levels by 30–40 % or more [2].

New treatment guidelines (*2013 ACC/AHA Guidelines on the Treatment of Blood Cholesterol to Reduce Atherosclerotic Cardiovascular Risk in Adults*) [3] for high cholesterol will likely double the number of Americans being prescribed these drugs, raising the number to a level which may exceed 70 million individuals in the US. This is particularly interesting in light of the fact that current research supports the view that the incidence of coronary heart disease (CHD) is essentially the same for people with elevated and normal blood serum cholesterol levels (see Chapter 15 on Cholesterol Screening).

The Cholesterol BRCT shown in the previous chapter suggests that the benefit from reducing cholesterol levels may not support the contention that cholesterol is a primary risk factor for CHD. Yet the people who take statins to lower their cholesterol do so in the hope of reducing their risk of heart disease.

Statins are certainly effective at reducing cholesterol levels. Doctors and researchers generally agree that statins also lower the incidence of CHD in individuals who have had heart attacks. However, it is not clear whether statins' heart benefits derive from lowering cholesterol or from something else they do in the body. On the other hand, does it really matter why statins work? Maybe cholesterol levels are not relevant—but so what? If statins reduce the incidence of CHD, should not everyone take them? After all, heart attacks are often deadly.

However, many of us are not going to die of a heart attack, or even experience CHD symptoms. Some of us have elevated cholesterol but no other risk factors for cardiovascular disease. Should we endure the cost and possible adverse effects of statins? Should we take a combination of drugs to continue to lower our blood serum cholesterol levels? What about swearing off tasty foods that are high in cholesterol? These are legitimate questions in spite of the continued focus on reducing cholesterol levels. Currently, opinions vary in the medical and scientific communities on the merits of prescribing statins to low risk populations [4, 5]. This continues to be a very controversial issue.

Before taking statins (or any drug for that matter), it is smart to do a little fact-finding. We must determine what these potent drugs do, what they do not do, and for whom. After all, even if they have benefits for some people, statins can cause side-effects and complications like rhabdomyolysis (muscle destruction); abnormal changes in liver function; myopathy (muscle disease); cataracts; adverse changes to memory, thinking, and concentration; depression and irritability; increased pain, tingling, and numbness; sleep problems; sexual dysfunction; blood sugar changes; and nausea. Some of these side effects can affect a significant number of people [6–10].

Statins may play a role in reducing inflammation and blood clots which may lead to reduced prevalence of CHD [11]. Statins can affect the innermost layer of cells lining our arteries (the endothelium), make smooth muscle cells less active, and affect the physiology of the artery wall [12]. A prominent scientist in this area states, "If the major benefits of statins are mediated through their effects on inflammation, thrombosis, and oxidation, we would also expect the relative benefits of statin therapy to be *independent* of baseline LDL cholesterol level." (Haywood et al. [13])

Indeed, if statins' primary benefits are a result of mechanisms unrelated to lowering LDL cholesterol levels, then we should focus more on the other risk factors for CHD. More resources should be allocated to clarify which conditions put people at the greatest risk for heart disease, and whether statins are effective against these conditions. Since our understanding is still incomplete, it is possible that millions of people are taking statins who should not be, and millions of people who should be, are not.

If cholesterol is not the primary controllable risk factor for CHD, then some people are unnecessarily bearing the cost and potential side effects of cholesterol-reducing drugs. But if statins are effective against something other than cholesterol, then individuals who could potentially benefit from taking statins are being overlooked. It looks like statins do many additional things in the body besides decreasing LDL cholesterol levels in the blood [14, 15].

A number of large, controlled, clinical trials with statins have been conducted involving tens of thousands of people. These clinical trials have included people without a history of CHD who take statins for *primary prevention* (individuals without previous CHD), as well as individuals with a history of CHD who take statins for *secondary prevention* (individuals with previous CHD). Results from these studies show that statins do reduce the incidence of cardiovascular events for both groups [16].

Diabetes, age, high blood pressure, smoking, family history, and even gender can all play a role in CHD, so these characteristics are called "risk factors." Many study participants have not one but multiple risk factors for CHD. But the risk factors vary from study to study, which makes it difficult to come to any meaningful conclusions about which patients will benefit from taking one or more specific statin drug.

Maybe people with diabetes will respond better to one drug, while smokers with high blood pressure will respond better to a different one. In other words, the uncertainty surrounding statin use remains high. However, one thing is clear: people who have already had a heart attack benefit significantly more from statins than people with no history of CHD.

Information in the Statin BRCTs came from a summary [16] that examined and compared the results of seven different studies. Four of them were major studies about the use of three statins (Zocor™, Lipitor™, and Pravachol™) by people without previous CHD. The other three studies investigated the use of the same three statins in populations with previous CHD. All of these clinical studies involved thousands of individuals with different sets of risk factors, lasted approximately 5 years, and provided data to calculate the cardiovascular benefits.

While the results can certainly be interpreted in a variety of ways, they provide a sense of the overall benefits from taking the three statins studied. The Statin BRCTs presented show the number of patients who benefited by taking statins for 5 years. The benefit was a decrease in cardiovascular events—heart attack or CHD death, depending on the study.

Primary Prevention Studies

The Statin BRCT shown in Fig. 16.1 represents individuals without previous CHD who have taken Zocor™, Lipitor™, or Pravacol™. The people who took statins experienced fewer cardiovascular events in comparison to the people who did not take statins. The darkened seats in each example represent the number of individuals without previous CHD who benefited from statin use, compared to people who didn't take statins.

In summary, in the primary prevention studies, between 16 and 43 out of 1,000 individuals without previous CHD benefited from taking statins over a 5-year period when compared to individuals not taking these drugs. The average of these studies is about 30, so approximately 30 out of 1,000 people benefited. In other words, the average absolute benefit rate for using the statins for primary prevention is about 3 % (3 out of 100). This means that the other 97 % of people taking statins for primary prevention did not benefit from taking these drugs, at least in terms of CHD.*

*__Primary Prevention__ A. *Heart Protection Study Group* (HPS) participants took Zocor™ (Simvastatin) and saw an absolute benefit of 43/1,000; **B.** *Collaborative Atorvastatin Diabetes Study* (CARDS) participants took Lipitor™ (Atorvastatin) and saw an absolute benefit of 40/1,000; **C.** *West of Scotland Coronary Prevention Study* (WOSCAPS) participants took Pravacol™ (Pravastatin) and saw an absolute benefit of 24/1,000; and **D.** *Anglo-Scandinavian Cardiac Outcomes Trial* (ASCOT) participants took Lipitor™ (Atorvastatin) and saw an absolute benefit of 16/1,000.

Secondary Prevention Studies

The Statin BRCT shown in Fig. 16.2 represents individuals with previous CHD who have taken Zocor™ or Lipitor™ or Pravacol™. The people who took statins experienced fewer cardiovascular events in comparison to the people who did not take the statins. The darkened seats in each example represent the number of people with previous CHD who benefited from statin use, compared to people not taking statins.

To summarize, for those people who had previous CHD, between 58 and 76 out of 1,000 individuals benefited from taking statins over a 5-year period when compared to those who did not take the drugs. The average of these studies is about 67, so approximately 67 out of 1,000 people benefited.

In other words, the absolute benefit rate from using the statins for secondary prevention is almost 7 %. Conversely, 93 % of the individuals in the studies did not benefit from taking the statins. Comparing Figs. 16.1 and 16.2, the benefits to individuals with previous heart attacks are clearly greater than the benefits for individuals with no previous CHD. The results** from these statin studies support the view that these drugs provide benefits greater than the benefits which would be achieved by lowering blood serum cholesterol levels. Based on the clinical trials shown in Fig. 16.2 about 7 % of these individuals could potentially benefit if they were all to take statins. As impressive as these benefits appear, individual decisions should not be based on nationwide benefit numbers.

Imagine that a patient is one of the approximately 180 million adult Americans who do not have any previous CHD. After his annual medical exam, he is told that everything is fine except his total blood serum cholesterol level is high at 245 mg. It is recommended that he should start taking a statin to lower his cholesterol. But it is also known that 1 person out of 1,000 will benefit from lowering his or her cholesterol to a "normal" level. Perhaps his blood serum cholesterol level does not warrant taking statins and the possible benefits of lowering his cholesterol with statins do not justify the costs, risks, and lifestyle changes.

However, statins could also have other benefits—benefits that may be more important than lowering cholesterol. Maybe these would tip the balance in favor of taking statins after all. So a doctor and patient need to evaluate the situation, consider the options, and make a decision based on a patient's level of acceptable risk.

Secondary Prevention A. *Scandinavian Simvastatin Survival Study Group* (4S) participants took Zocor™ (Simvastatin) and saw an absolute benefit of 76,1,000, **B.** *Pravastatin or Atorvastatin Evaluation and Infection Therapy* (PROVE-IT) participants took Lipitor™ (Atorvastatin) and saw an absolute benefit of 66,1,000, and **C.** *Heart Protection Study* (HPS) participants took Zocor™ (Simvastatin) and saw an absolute benefit of 58/1,000.

References

1. Herper, M. (2013). As statins soar, use of other cholesterol medicines declines. *Forbes, Pharma & Health* 10 May. www.forbes.com/sites/matthewherper/2013/05/29/as-statins-soar-use-of-other-cholesterol-medicines-declines/
2. Fuhrmans ,V. (2001). European panel to conduct review of cholesterol drugs. *Wall Street Journal* New York, 10 August.
3. CarStone, N. J., Robinson, J., Lichtenstein, A. H., Bairey Merz, C. N., Lloyd-Jones, D. M., Blum, C. B., McBride, P., Eckel, R. H., Schwartz, J. S., Goldberg, A. C., Shero, S. T., Gordon, D., Smith, S. C., Jr., Levy, D., Watson, K., & Wilson, P. W. (2013). ACC/AHA guideline on the treatment of blood cholesterol to reduce atherosclerotic cardiovascular risk in adults: A report of the American College of Cardiology/American Heart Association Task Force on Practice Guidelines. *Journal of the American College of Cardiology, 63*(25 Pt B), 2889–2934.
4. Center for Science in the Public Interest (2004) Washington. (released 23 Sept. 2004, accessed Oct. 2006). http://www.cspinet.org/new/200409231.html.

5. Therapeutics Initiative (2003) Do statins have a role in primary prevention? University of British Columbia, Vancouver. (released 16 Oct. 2003, accessed Oct. 2006). http://www.ti.ubc.ca/pages/letter48.htm.

6. Golomb, B. A., & Criqui, M. H. (2006). *Statin adverse effects. university of California San Diego Statin effects study group.* (updated 2 Aug. 2006, accessed Oct. 2006). http://medicine.ucsd.edu/SES/statin_information.htm.

7. Talbert, R. L. (2006). Safety issues with statin therapy. *Journal of the American Pharmaceutical Association, 46*(4), 479–488.

8. Hippisley-Cox, J., & Coupland, C. (2010). Unintended effects of statins in men and women in England and wales: Population based cohort study using the Q research database. *British Medical Journal 340*, Article ID: c2197.

9. El-Salem, K., Ababneh, B., Rudnicki, S., Malkawi, A., Alrefai, A., Khader, Y., Saadeh, R., & Saydam, M. (2011). Prevalence and risk factors of muscle complications secondary to statins. *Muscle and Nerve, 44*(6), 877–881. doi:10.1002/mus.22205.

10. Vinogradova, Y., Coupland, C., & Hippisley-Cox, J. (2011). Exposure to statins and risk of common cancers: a series of nested case-control studies. *BMC Cancer, 11*(1), 409. doi:10.1186/1471-2407-11-409.

11. Liao, J. K., & Laufs, U. (2005). Pleiotropic effects of statins. *Annual Review Pharmcology and Toxicology, 45*, 89–118.

12. Kolovou, G. (2001). The treatment of coronary heart disease: an update: Part 3: Statins beyond cholesterol lowering. *Current Medical Research and Opinion, 17*(1), 34–37.

13. Hayward, R. A., Hofer, T. P., & Vijan, S. (2006). Narrative review: Lack of evidence for recommended low-density lipoprotein treatment targets: A solvable problem. *Annals of Internal Medicine, 145*(7), 520–530.

14. Vaughan, C. J., Murphy, M. B., & Buckley, B. M. (1996). Statins do more than just lower cholesterol. *Lancet, 348*(9034), 1079–1082.

15. Massy, Z. A., Keane, W. F., & Kasiske, B. L. (1996). Inhibition of the mevalonate pathway: Benefits beyond cholesterol reduction? *Lancet, 347*(8994), 102–103.

16. Regier, L. (2006). Personal communication, Saskatoon City Hospital, 701 Queen St., Saskatoon, Sk Canada S7K0M7. See also NNTs for statins in variable risk groups – major trial data (standardized for 5 years), Table 1. Available online at http://www.rxfiles.ca/acrobat/Lipid-Q&A-Update-Oct04.pdf.

Chapter 17
Annual Exam

Mr. W came to the office for his annual exam. He was a healthy 72-year-old man with high blood pressure and some mild aches and pains. He had recently retired as an engineer, but remained active, although was not an avid exerciser. He took two medicines for his blood pressure and saw me one other time a year to have it checked. He also took a few supplements, which varied from month to month based on which pills his wife put in his hands every morning. He never had chest pains or shortness of breath, and he woke up once a night to urinate and had some increased frequency, but it was nothing that disturbed him. And his weight had been stable. He had been receiving colonoscopies regularly, and on one occasion had a few polyps removed. He had a normal scope three years ago, but his GI doctor suggested he come back for another one in 5 years. He did check PSA's with his Urologist and did see a Cardiologist as well, although I could not ascertain why. In fact, every few years he had a stress test, echocardiogram, and carotid ultrasound by that doctor.

Today he wanted "the works," just to make sure he was healthy. Of course he expected blood work, and he had come in fasting. He thought it may be a good idea to check an EKG, since we had not done one in a while. And he wanted to give me a urine specimen. Also he knew it was time to do a thorough exam, not the cursory looking-over that I typically gave him.

"Check everything out," he said. "Even the finger up the rear end. And my wife says make sure to listen to my neck, so I don't get a stroke."

I asked him what he wanted to look for in the blood. "Diabetes, cholesterol, everything," he said. "And my wife says to check my thyroid too, because I can't lose weight. And all the vitamin levels."

In the past he had tests for cholesterol that were not remarkably elevated and, after discussion of treatment risks, and benefits, he decided not to take statins. He had no symptoms suggestive of thyroid disease or diabetes, and no change in his urine that might cause alarms. I talked to him briefly about the risks and benefit of some of the exams and tests he requested, but he did not seem deterred by my reservations, especially my concern about the potential high risk of false positive results.

© Springer International Publishing Switzerland 2015
E. Rifkin, A. Lazris, *Interpreting Health Benefits and Risks*,
DOI 10.1007/978-3-319-11544-3_17

"If you find something, then we can decide what to do about it," he said. "But there's no harm in looking."

I took my questioning a step further, just to see how aggressive he wanted me to be. "If I hear a noise in your neck it could indicate you have a blockage of your carotid artery, although the exam is so inaccurate that chances are it is not blocked. And even if you have a blockage that does not mean you're necessarily more prone to a stroke. But it does mean I have to do more testing to figure it out."

"I'm ok with more tests."

"Let's say we find a 70 % blockage. Do we fix it, even though we're not sure leaving it alone will cause you to have a stroke, and even though surgery to fix it can itself cause a stroke?"

"I don't want that. We can keep an eye on it. It will make me feel better knowing what's going on. Maybe that will give me the push I need to lose weight and do some walking. But you know, I don't want surgery unless I'm at the edge of death. I just want all the information."

With that in mind, I examined Mr. W, and we sent him for a few less tests than he originally had requested, but tests that both he and I felt would be safe and would give him the information he craved.

A. Key Questions

- Does a patient need an annual physical? What will be covered there that is not typically discussed during other visits?
- Does a patient want an annual physical? If so, what is he/she looking to achieve?
- Which physical exam components are potentially effective in a patient that may reveal problems and improve health outcome? Are there harms?
- Which labs tests and studies are potentially helpful for a patient? What is the likelihood of false positive and negative tests, and how effective are these tests in finding fixable problems that improve clinical outcome?

B. Risks and Benefits

- **There is no evidence that an annual exam impacts outcome. A recent study showed a statistically insignificant drop in total mortality of 6/1,000, but an increase in cardiac mortality of 7/1,000 in people getting annual exams over a decade. There were 200/1,000 more diagnoses charted for those people who had the exam compared to those who did not (Fig. 17.1).**
- **Annual blood work has a low diagnostic value, adding information in 7–30/1,000 tests based on which test is ordered. The false positive rate is as high as 360/1,000 (Fig. 17.2).** Therefore approximately 10 out of 1,000 lab tests

will demonstrate something clinically important, while 360 out of 1,000 labs tests will be falsely abnormal and not be of any clinical value. Many of the latter can lead to unnecessary testing and treatment that can cause harm and false disease labeling.

- Annual urine tests have no proven benefit in reducing death from bladder cancer, but have a false positive rate of 900/1,000, and lead to a large number of unnecessary tests.

- **Rectal exams have a false positive rate of approximately 700/1,000 for both prostate cancer and rectal cancer. In addition there is a high false negative rate: 250/1,000 people with prostate cancer had a normal prostate exam. There is no meaningful change in mortality in those who get rectal exams (Fig.** 17.3**).** Therefore, the vast majority of abnormal rectal exams do not indicate the presence of disease, often leading to unnecessary testing, while a large number of normal rectal exams occur in people who actually do have significant disease.

- Exams for abdominal aneurysms (AAA) have a 500/1,000 false positive rate, and 500/1,000 people with significant aneurysms had a normal exam. Therefore, an abnormal exam has a 50 % chance of occurring in a person without disease, often leading to unnecessary testing, while people with significant AAA have a 50 % chance of having a normal exam, leading to false reassurance. There is no proven change in mortality by performing the exam.

- Exams for carotid bruits have a high false positive and negative rate and have not been shown to reduce the incidence of stroke or death. Apparently, 5/1,000 people with bruits have clinically meaningful carotid disease, and there is a high rate of unnecessary testing due to false positive rate. Also, 500/1,000 people with significant carotid disease do not have detectable bruits, and thus the absence of a bruit does not rule out the presence of significant disease.

- Routine EKG testing has a false positive rate of 400–750/1,000, and that number is highest in older patients. It is a poor predictor of adverse events (1–7/1,000 people with abnormal tests have cardiac events in a year), even in the preoperative setting. The false positive rate can lead to unnecessary and potentially harmful testing, can lead to false disease labeling, and can delay surgery when done as part of a pre-operative exam.

- Skin exams have not been shown to reduce mortality from skin cancer and have a high false positive rate (72–975/1,000 depending on the type of cancer), leading to many unnecessary biopsies. As many as 200/1,000 older patients who have skin biopsies have adverse effects, and there is little evidence that detecting and removing non-melanoma skin cancers in the elderly impacts mortality or quality of life.

- A VA panel recommended that periodic weights, blood pressure checks, and (when appropriate) pap smears do have value. There may be other value in an annual exam that is more difficult to quantify, such as a discussion between doctor and patient about various health matters, medicines, and screening tests.

BRCTs:
Annual Exam

The Benefits of an Annual Exam

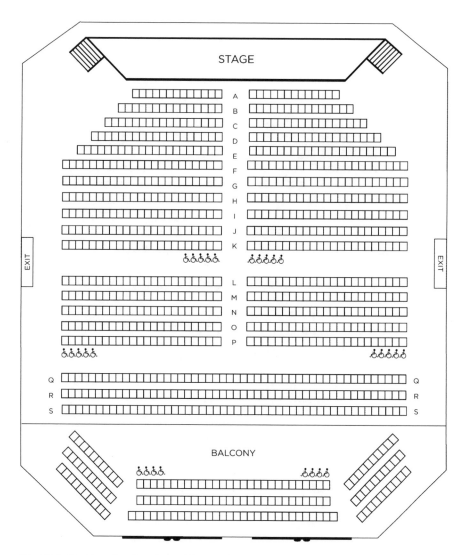

Fig. 17.1 The Benefits of an Annual Exam. If 1,000 people sitting in a theater have an annual exam, none, represented by no blackened seats, will have any statistically significant improvement in health outcome or mortality

Accuracy of Annual Blood Tests in Finding Disease

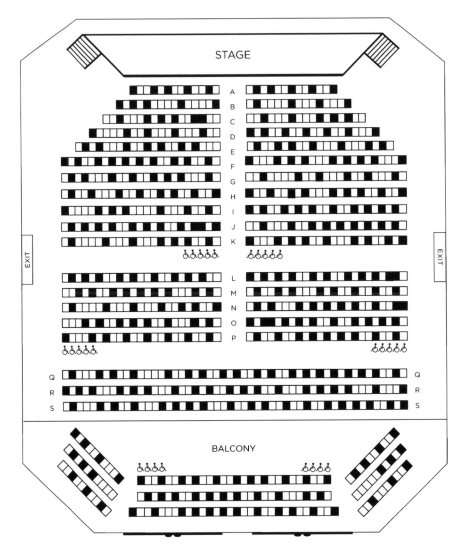

Fig. 17.2 Accuracy of Annual Blood Tests in Finding Disease. Out of 1,000 screening blood tests performed as part of an annual exam, approximately 360 will show false positive abnormalities, represented by blackened seats, that are not indicative of any disease process. Routine urine testing yields a false positive rate of 900/1,000 tests, which is higher than the number of seats blocked. Approximately 7–30 out of 1,000 routine labs add some clinical information that may be of value

Benefits of a Rectal and Prostate Exam

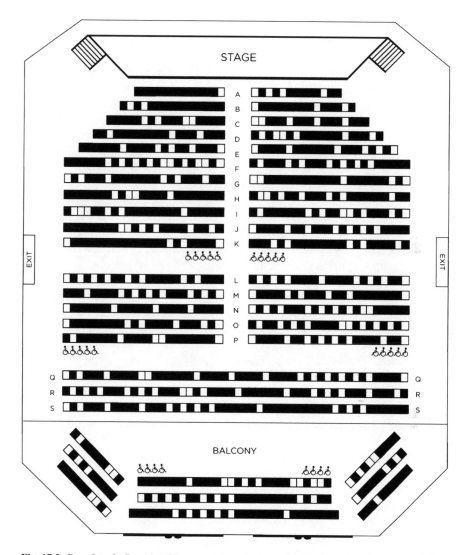

Fig. 17.3 Benefits of a Rectal and Prostate Exam. Of 1,000 people sitting in a theater who have a rectal exam as part of the annual exam and have an abnormality detected either in the prostate or rectum, 700 of them will be false positives, represented by blackened seats, and will often need further testing to prove that they are benign

C. Discussion

Annual physical exams are a mainstay of modern American medical practice. They constitute a crucial mission of primary care, and they are viewed by the community at large as beneficial and even necessary for the promotion of good health. It has been estimated that 44 million Americans receive an annual exam every year at a cost of $8 billion annually.[1,2] In fact, annual exams comprise 80/1,000 of all physician visits. Patients want and expect an exam. One study suggested that, like with Mr. W, the exam and subsequent annual testing may decrease patient worry, as well as providing a forum to discuss health issues not related to a patient's specific medical problems or complaints [1]. Doctors also largely encourage the annual physical. In a 2005 survey, more than half of doctors stated support for preventive exams and tests, even those that had been deemed to be ineffective [2].

What specifically comprises an annual exam will vary between doctors and patients. The one constant is that the tests ordered, and the physical exam performed, are not driven by specific health concerns or complaints that the patient may express. Symptom-based exams and testing fall into a different category. The annual exam is a forum to look for problems about which the patient may be unaware. It is essentially a preventive visit; if we can find problems before they become severe, it is argued, then we may be able to improve outcome. But by fishing for problems, we may uncover false positives: Abnormal results that are not reflective of real disease. It is felt that for 14 aspects of a typical annual exam, including tests and labs, there is a 500/1,000 chance of finding at least one false positive.[3] Since may lab panels themselves have more than 14 tests, then a comprehensive annual exam can potentially reveal many false positives, which could lead to over testing and overtreatment. There is also a danger of false negatives, where tests or exams are normal in the face of real disease, a situation that sows a sense of false security.

Several common elements of the annual exam have been studied. These include blood tests, urine tests, the EKG, aspects of the physical exam, and gynecological tests. Many screening tests that are often discussed at an annual exam have been covered in other chapters, including mammograms, stress tests, colonoscopies, cholesterol screening, and smoking cessation. We will focus on other aspects of the annual exam to ascertain what evidence exists for benefit or harm.

A VA panel evaluated various aspects of the physical exam using available evidence. They concluded that certain parts of the exam were medically sensible, such as periodic weights, blood pressure check every 2 years, and pap smears every 3 years for sexually active women under age 65 who have a cervix. They found no

[1] http://well.blogs.nytimes.com/2013/01/21/a-check-on-physicals/?_php=true&_type=blogs&_r=0.
[2] http://www.slate.com/articles/health_and_science/medical_examiner/2013/08/annual_checkups_going_to_the_doctor_when_you_re_not_sick_does_more_harm.html.
[3] http://www.slate.com/articles/health_and_science/medical_examiner/2013/08/annual_checkups_going_to_the_doctor_when_you_re_not_sick_does_more_harm.html.

evidence to support exams of the prostate, carotid arteries, abdomen to assess the presence of an aneurysm, lung, pulse, lymph nodes, and the peripheral nerves, all of which have high false positive and false negative rates. There is also no evidence that a routine exam of the heart will yield useful clinical information that would not otherwise be obtained in a patient's history (most notably the presence of murmurs that may indicate valvular heart disease, a condition typically only treated when symptoms occur), or that checking a pulse for arrhythmias such as atrial fibrillation will yield clinically useful information. The study concluded: "Comprehensive routine physical examinations are not recommended for the asymptomatic adult."[4][3] The US Preventive Services Task Force evaluates many parts of the annual exam, but does not comment on the benefits or risks of the exam itself. The most salient barrier that precludes a sensible discussion of the exam and its various parts is the lack of good evidence to demonstrate the ramifications of screening on mortality and morbidity over an extended period of time.[5]

One large meta-analysis recently evaluated the annual exam as a whole. Fourteen studies comprising 180,000 people compared those who had annual exams to those who did not over a 10-year period. Most annual visits included vital signs, a comprehensive physical exam, EKG, and multiple lab tests including cholesterol. Overall, those in the annual exam arm had an increase in the number of diagnoses made by 200/1,000 compared to those who did not have a yearly visit. However, over 9–10 years, there was no statistically significant difference in mortality, cardiac mortality, cancer mortality, hospitalization, morbidity, or disability [4].

Annual Routine Blood Tests: Blood tests are part of most exams. Several organizations cite the utility of cholesterol screening, which we have discussed in another chapter. In one older study, the diagnostic value of a test was defined as its ability to detect a new clinical diagnosis, although the authors did not comment on whether such detection led to treatment, better outcomes, or harm. Overall there was diagnostic value of 28/1,000 chemistry panels ordered, 9/1,000 complete blood counts (CBC), and 7/1,000 thyroid tests. There were many false positives, with overall 360/1,000 tests demonstrating an abnormality, and 31/1,000 requiring further testing to prove that nothing was wrong [5].

A study looking only at CBC found that 5/1,000 led to a treatable diagnosis, and 25/1,000 required further testing to prove they were normal [6]. The USPSTF suggests that there is no compelling evidence to recommend thyroid testing due to a high rate of false positives and a possible danger of over treating clinically insignificant abnormal thyroid tests. Overall they suggest that screening may identify 3/1,000 people with hypothyroidism over 5 years, but that treatment efficacy for such people has not been determined, so they may receive thyroid medicines unnecessarily.[6]

---

[4] http://www.ncbi.nlm.nih.gov/books/NBK82767.

[5] http://www.acpinternist.org/archives/2010/01/annual.htm.

[6] http://www.uspreventiveservicestaskforce.org/3rduspstf/thyroid/thyrrs.htm.

The Routine Urinalysis: Many patients request an annual urinalysis, primarily as a means of detecting small amounts of blood that could portend bladder cancer. The American Cancer Society suggests that most studies do not demonstrate a higher rate of clinically significant bladder cancer detection with urinalysis, primarily because most people with even early treatable bladder cancer will have sufficient bleeding to be visually observed.[7] The USPSTF also recommends against bladder cancer screening, citing a 900/1,000 false positive rate of a routine urinalysis. While there is no evidence that early detection of bladder cancer will improve outcome, there is a potential for harm from urinalysis, as many people with positive tests will be subjected to a cystoscopic evaluation, which itself carries a 25/1,000 risk of bleeding or perforation of the bladder.[8]

The Rectal Exam: Often patients and doctors consider a finger probe of the rectum to be a painful necessity of the exam, especially in men. The goal of that exam is to detect rectal cancer and, in men, prostate cancer. There have been a few case–control studies that suggest a tiny reduction in prostate cancer mortality among men who undergo regular screening, but those findings have been inconsistent, and the lack of abnormalities on a prostate exam does not imply the absence of cancer. In fact, in one study 250/1,000 of men who presented with metastatic prostate cancer had had normal rectal exams[9][7]. An ongoing study in prostate screening that encompasses both rectal exam and PSA (which is covered elsewhere in the book) reported its 7-year findings showing a prostate cancer mortality decrease of only 0.3/10,000 in the screened men [8].

The rectal exam also is plagued by a high rate of false positives and a low sensitivity, like many other screening tests. The false positive rate (abnormal exams in patients who, after further testing, had no disease) for prostate cancer is 720/1,000, and for rectal cancer it is 700/1,000. Also, as mentioned, rectal exams have a high false negative rate; 410/1,000 and 240/1,000 prostate and rectal cancers, respectively, are missed in people with normal exams [9, 10]. Many men with false positive screens will be subjected to prostate biopsies or colonoscopies, which are not without risk. Others with false positive exams will be inappropriately labeled as having disease. Also, there is continuing controversy as to whether diagnosing prostate cancer by screening will reduce prostate cancer mortality as previously discussed, an important consideration especially given the significant morbidity of prostate cancer treatments.

Aneurysm Screening: Abdominal Aortic Aneurysms (AAA) are weak areas of the largest artery in our body that, if they become too large, can burst, causing a significant mortality rate. They typically present without symptoms, so many people suggest screening for AAA in the annual exam. The physical exam for AAA is done

---

[7] http://www.cancer.org/cancer/bladdercancer/detailedguide/bladder-cancer-detection.

[8] http://www.uspreventiveservicestaskforce.org/uspstf11/bladdercancer/bladcanes.pdf.

[9] http://www.cancer.gov/cancertopics/pdq/screening/prostate/HealthProfessional/page3#Reference3.14.

with a stethoscope on the abdomen in a search for bruits. Overall the diagnostic yield of the exam is poor; the false positive rate exceeds 500/1,000, and more than 500/1,000 of aneurysms cannot be detected on exam.[11] The USPSTF recommends one-time ultrasound screening for AAA in male smokers between the ages of 65 and 75 where the risk of having a clinically large aneurysm is approximately 50/1,000. However, there is no evidence that such screening has any impact on overall mortality, and it could lead to overtreatment with surgery, which itself has a mortality of 50/1,000 and a severe morbidity of 300/1,000. Screening is not recommended in other groups where the incidence of AAA is far lower.[10]

Carotid Artery Screening: Very often doctors listen to the carotid arteries to find bruits that may be caused by a narrowing of the artery. Strokes can be caused by blocked carotid arteries, many of which are asymptomatic. Therefore it is felt that bruits may indicate serious carotid disease that, if found early, can be treated before instigating a stroke. Several studies have suggested that the incidence of bruits on exam increases the risk of stroke in that patient by 6/1,000 per year, although such a finding does not add any prognostic information to the patient's overall risk factors for stroke. Also, the presence of a bruit does not predict where the patient may have a stroke; often the stroke occurs in the opposite side of the brain than where the bruit is found [12].

In fact, most bruits are false positives, with 750/1,000 of bruits not corresponding to carotid stenoses and thus not putting the patient at risk of having a stroke. Of all people with bruits, only 5/1,000 have significant carotid disease. Also the test has poor sensitivity, as approximately half of patients with significant carotid disease do not have bruits [13]. Typically, if a bruit is heard, patients will be sent for carotid ultrasound or MRA, which in turn can lead to even more invasive testing since those procedures themselves have a high false positive rate (see chapter on carotid screening). Since 40/1,000 patients have bruits, carotid auscultation can lead to a significant amount of over-testing if performed as part of a general exam given its high false positive rate, as well as giving many people without bruits false assurance that they do not have significant stenosis given its high false negative rate. Both scenarios may lead to as much or more harm than benefit.

EKG Screening: We have discussed EKG tests to some extent in the stress test chapter. Several studies do suggest that an EKG can help predict adverse cardiac outcomes. One older study found that in men there was a 1/1,000 increased risk of cardiac death per year with minor EKG abnormalities, and a 7/1,000 increased risk with major abnormalities. In women these numbers were 1/1,000 and 5/1,000 respectively.[14] The USPSTF recommends against using resting or stress EKG screening in low risk patients and defers from making any judgment in higher risk patients due to a paucity of evidence that such tests improve cardiac outcome. There are not studies that suggest that any subsequent testing or intervention after an abnormal EKG will lead to benefit or harm.

---

[10] http://www.uspreventiveservicestaskforce.org/uspstf/uspsaneu.htm.

The false positive and false negative rates of EKG testing are very high; normal tests do not accurately predict those who are safe from cardiac complications, while abnormal tests frequently occur in people at low risk for cardiac disease, something that may lead to unnecessary and possibly harmful additional testing.[11] A study done in athletes showed that the false positive rate of abnormal EKG's approximated 400/1,000 [15]. Also, in studies looking at the value of EKG's used for preoperative evaluation, a common practice in health care today, the EKG failed to predict those patients who were vulnerable to a poor cardiac outcome beyond what the rest of the history prognosticated. Most striking in these studies was that 440/1,000 patients without cardiac problems had abnormal EKG's, and that number was 750/1,000 in the elderly [16–18]. Therefore, abnormalities on screening EKG's are common, are poorly predictive of adverse outcome, may lead to interventions that are unnecessary and harmful, but do identify a small number of people at risk for cardiac death whose underlying history often also provides similar prognostic information.

Skin Cancer Screening: Often in their annual physicals patients receive a total skin exam or are referred to a dermatologist to do the same. Every year 2–4 million Americans are diagnosed with non-melanoma skin cancers (squamous cell and basal cell), the vast majority of which are not fatal. Approximately, 75,000 are diagnosed with melanoma, with an annual mortality rate of 9,700. The USPSTF suggests that such exams are not clinically effective. While skin exams may discover melanomas earlier, there is no evidence that such early detection improves mortality or morbidity. Also the discovery of non-melanoma skin cancers is of moot value in many cases, in that they often have little potential for mortality or morbidity if left alone, especially in the elderly.

The National Cancer Institute cites one poorly performed study that compares a large cohort of patients in a skin screening program with a non-screened population and finds a reduction in melanoma mortality of 1/100,000 over 10 years. The skin exam also has a very high false positive rate, finding moles and lesions that, after biopsy, were determined not to be cancer. In fact, 975/1,000 lesions felt to be melanoma by skin exam were proved to be benign moles after biopsy, 72/1,000 feared squamous cell cancer were benign, and 193/1,000 feared basal cell cancers were benign.[12, 13] Such a high false positive rate, coupled with the doubt about the efficacy of removing non-melanoma cancer in many circumstances, leads to a large number of unnecessary biopsies and surgeries for lesions and cancers discovered by skin exam that are not dangerous. One study of the elderly suggests that 200/1,000 of people who underwent skin biopsies suffered significant complications, without deriving benefit.[14] Like with many aspects of the annual exam, there seems to be a large chance of harm occurring from over-diagnosis, with little evidence of benefit from a skin exam.

---

[11] http://www.uspreventiveservicestaskforce.org/uspstf11/coronarydis/chdupd.htm#results.

[12] http://www.uspreventiveservicestaskforce.org/uspstf09/skincancer/skincanrs.htm.

[13] http://www.cancer.gov/cancertopics/pdq/screening/skin/HealthProfessional/page2.

[14] www.ucsf.edu/news/2013/04/105436/surgery-nonfatal-skin-cancers-might-not-be-best-elderly-patients.

References

1. Boulware, L. E., et al. (2007). Systematic review: The value of the periodic health evaluation. *Annals of Internal Medicine, 146,* 289–300.
2. Prochazka, A. V., et al. (2005). Support of evidence-based guidelines for the annual physical examination: A survey of primary care providers. *Archives of Internal Medicine, 165,* 1347–1352.
3. Bloomfield, H., & Wilt, T. (2011). Evidence brief: Role of the annual comprehensive physical examination in the asymptomatic adult, VA Evidence-based Synthesis Program Evaluation Briefs, October, 2011.
4. Krogsboll, L., et al. (2012). General health checks in adults for reducing morbidity and mortality from disease. *British Medical Journal, 345,* 7191.
5. Boland, B. J., et al. (1996). Yield of laboratory tests for case finding in the ambulatory general exam. *American Journal of Medicine, 101*(2), 141–152.
6. Ruttimann, S., et al. (1992). Usefulness of complete blood count as a case finding tool in medical outpatients. *Annals of Internal Medicine, 116*(1), 44–50.
7. Otto, S., & Roobol, M. (2006). Case control studies in evaluating prostate cancer screening: An overview. *European Association of Urology, 4,* 219–227.
8. Andriole, G., et al. (2009). Mortality results from a randomized prostate cancer screening trial. *New England Journal of Medicine, 360,* 1310–1319.
9. Ang, C. W., et al. (2008). The diagnostic value of a digital rectal exam in primary care for palpable rectal tumors. *Colorectal Disease, 10*(8), 789–792.
10. Buntinx, F., et al. (1994). The diagnostic value of digital rectal exam in primary care screening for prostate cancer. *Family Practice, 16*(6), 621–626.
11. Pysklywec, M., & Evans, M. (2009). Diagnosing abdominal aortic aneurysm: How good is the physical exam?". *Canadian Family Physician, 45,* 2069–2070.
12. Aronson, L., & Landenfeld, C. (1998). Examining older people for carotid bruits. *Journal of General Internal Medicine, 13*(2), 140–141.
13. Ratchford, E. V., et al. (2009). Carotid bruit for detection of hemodynamically significant carotid stenosis: The northern Manhattan study. *Neurological Research, 31*(7), 748–752.
14. De Bacquer, D., et al. (1998). Prognostic value of ECG findings for total, cardiovascular, and coronary heart disease death in men and women. *Heart, 1998*(80), 570–577.
15. Pelliccia, A., et al. (2000). Clinical significance of abnormal ECG patterns in trained athletes. *Circulation, 102,* 278–284.
16. Noordzij, P. G., et al. (2006). Prognostic value of routine preoperative electrocardiography in patients undergoing noncardiac surgery. *American Journal of Cardiology, 97,* 1103–1106.
17. Liu, L. L., et al. (2002). Preoperative electrocardiogram abnormalities do not predict postoperative cardiac complications in geriatric surgical patients. *Journal of American Geriatrics Society, 50,* 1186–1191.
18. Van Klei, W. A., et al. (2007). The value of routine preoperative electrocardiography in predicting myocardial infarction after noncardiac surgery. *Annals of Surgery, 246,* 165–170.

Chapter 18
Screening for and Treating Dementia

Mr. N had been married for 60 years to his wife. Over the past several years her memory declined and she was diagnosed with Alzheimer's Dementia. He brought her to several neurologists after the diagnosis was made. She had CT scans, MRI tests, and even an EEG to see if she was perhaps having asymptomatic seizures. Several of these tests were repeated more than once. She had copious lab tests, none of which revealed a definitive cause that could be treated.

She could be very forgetful, and her symptoms varied from day to day. She had total denial that she had any memory issues and berated her husband when he suggested it. She fought him even when he tried to help her. At times she insisted people had visited her, although they had long been deceased. On occasion she insisted that they were supposed to be somewhere, refusing to believe otherwise. She sometimes forgot to use the toilet properly, dressed improperly, and refused to eat. She had lost some weight. She soiled her clothes. And she had walked out of the house and gotten lost.

From the start, Mrs. N's doctors tried various medicines that might help her disease. She went on Aricept™ for a few weeks, but developed nausea and refused to continue. She then tried an Exelon™ patch. At first Mr. N believed that may have helped her mood a bit, as she was less inclined to talk back to him, but he saw very little else of promise. Her doctor then added a medicine called Namenda™ to the patch. Again, Mr. N thought that perhaps he saw some improvement in her behavior, and her neurologist noted a slight improvement on her memory test. But over time, as her disease continued to progress, he was convinced that neither medicine had really made a meaningful dent in her disease.

"Can we just stop these drugs and see where she ends up?" he asked me. Mr. N did not believe in using medicines that had no purpose. "One of my friends told me that if we stop them and she gets worse, then she'll never get as good as she is now."

I told him that if we stopped the pills, one at a time, then he could see if she was really benefiting from them. If she worsened off the pills, then we could restart them. Since these pills had no impact on the disease itself, and only mitigated the symptoms, there was no harm in stopping them and then adding them back if

© Springer International Publishing Switzerland 2015
E. Rifkin, A. Lazris, *Interpreting Health Benefits and Risks*,
DOI 10.1007/978-3-319-11544-3_18

needed. I also showed him the available evidence regarding the efficacy of the drugs. Since, unlike other interventions, the success of Alzheimer's drugs was measured by varied memory tests that did not always translate well into clinical relevant endpoints, the data I gave him hardly helped him make a decision.

I explained that he would have to decide if his wife declined off the medicines. There was nothing more objective on which we could rely. I reiterated that no medicine available changed the disease's course, and that unless he saw a clinically significant change then she was no better on the medicines than off. It was also clear from the data that I showed him that the bulk of improvement occurred in the first six months of drug administration, and after that time patients progressed at the same rate as if they were not taking any medicines. After some thought, he decided to try to taper off the medicines, starting with Namenda™, which was far more expensive.

A. Key Questions

- In people with memory loss is there any benefit to screen for various causes of dementia? Is it important to label the type of dementia precisely? Are there down sides of screening?
- Is the patient someone who may benefit from a trial of Alzheimer's Drugs? Which symptoms are expected to improve?
- Will the drugs have any impact on the disease outcome, and will symptom improvement persist for a prolonged period?
- What side effects can occur, and what should the patients do if they experience any of the side effects? How common are the side effects?
- Are there differences between the various drugs available on the market? If one does not work, is it worth trying another? Is there benefit in combining drugs?
- Can the drugs be stopped if either they do not seem to be working or if they have been used for a long time and the clinical benefit is questionable? What are the possible adverse outcomes if the drug is stopped suddenly?

B. Risks and Benefits

- **Testing for causes of memory loss reveals approximately 3/1,000 people whose memory loss can be fully reversed with treatment of findings (Fig. 18.1).**
- Dementia drugs can potentially control symptoms but do not impact the course of the disease. Most studies base drug efficacy on the results of dementia tests rather than clinical parameters.
- There is little to no difference between the various dementia drugs, especially those in the cholinesterase inhibitor category. Memantine (Namenda™) does have different properties and seems less effective for early disease.

- There is no evidence that combining drugs leads to any enhanced benefit.
- Overall in studies of dementia drugs there are approximately 300/1,000 patients in the placebo group who exhibit significant improvement. Therefore, there is a very strong placebo effect.
- **Approximately 92/1,000 people who take dementia drugs have some degree of improvement over placebo for up to a year, although typically the improvement levels off after a few months (Fig.** 18.2)**.**
- **An excess of 70/1,000 people who take dementia drugs over placebo have severe gastrointestinal reactions prompting withdrawal from studies. There is also an excess rate of more serious side effects including syncope (13/1,000) and hip fracture (2.2/1,000) (Fig.** 18.3)**.**
- There is no evidence that stopping dementia drugs leads to serious consequences.

BRCTs:
Screening for and Treating Dementia

Screening for Dementia

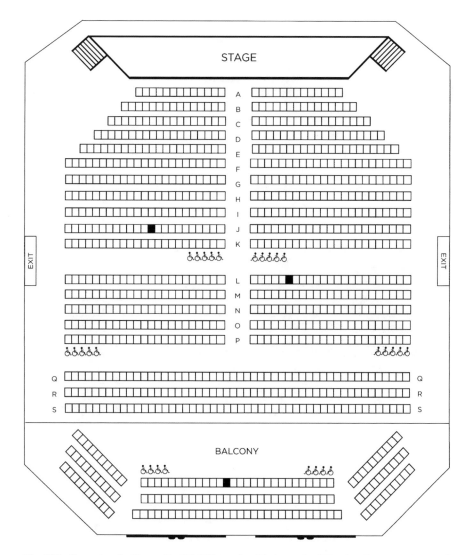

Fig. 18.1 Screening for Dementia. If 1,000 people with dementia sitting in a theater are screened with testing, approximately 3 of them, represented by blackened seats, will have ailments discovered that, when treated, can fully reverse their dementia

The Efficacy of Dementia Drugs

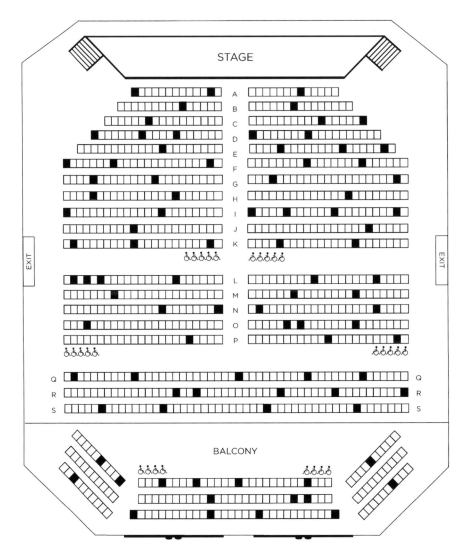

Fig. 18.2 The Efficacy of Dementia Drugs. Approximately 92 out of 1,000 people sitting in a theater, represented by blackened seats, with dementia have some measurable improvement for up to a year if they take dementia drugs compared to those who take placebo. The improvement may be very small and is typically discovered by testing and not by caregiver evaluation. There is very little difference between drugs, and there is no additive effect

Side effects of Dementia Drugs

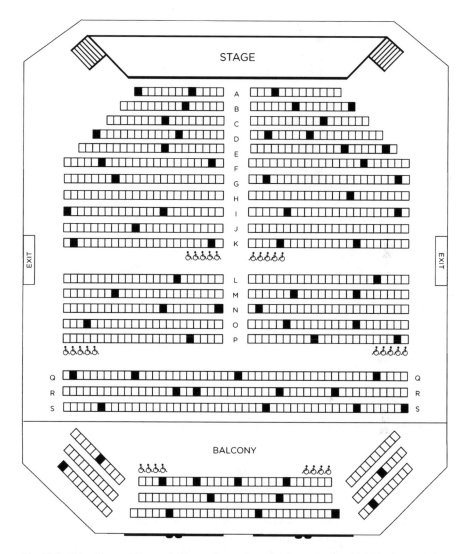

Fig. 18.3 Side effects of Dementia Drugs. Approximately 70 people out of 1,000 who are sitting in a theater, represented by blackened seats, and who receive dementia drugs will experience significant gastrointestinal side effects compared to 1,000 who receive placebo. These side effects typically cause people to stop taking the drugs. A smaller number of people, 2–13 out of 1,000 who take the drugs, have more severe side effects compared to those who take placebo, including hip fracture and complete heart block

C. Discussion

Alzheimer's disease is a condition of brain cell degeneration whose cause is unknown. Currently Alzheimer's cannot be diagnosed by testing. Many other forms of progressive dementia differ somewhat from Alzheimer's and thus acquire unique diagnostic names (Frontotemporal dementia, Lewy Body dementia, Parkinson's dementia, Vascular dementia), but most similarly cause brain deterioration, memory loss, and cognitive decline. Alzheimer's is the sixth leading cause of death in the country and is found in half of all people over the age of 85. Currently it is estimated that 5.3 million people are inflicted with the disease. The ultimate course of Alzheimer's patients is loss of speech, inability to carry out activities of daily living, loss of recognition, erratic behavior, and the inability to sensibly interact with the world around them [1].

Before treating dementia, many doctors screen patients with various tests to determine if treatable forms of memory loss exist that would be amenable to curative treatment. These could include NPH (normal pressure hydrocephalus), an accumulation of fluid in the brain ventricles; hypothyroidism; infections; tumor; and low vitamin B12 levels. Doctors may order brain scans, labs tests, neurological evaluations, EEG tests, and depression screens as part of this process. A meta-analysis suggests that while up to 90/1,000 people with dementia may be found to have a reversible etiology when tested, only 3/1,000 actually fully reversed with treatment [2]. Thus, even after screening is completed, and various causes of the memory loss were treated, 997/1,000 patients still had memory loss and signs of dementia.

There are various means of screening patients for the presence of dementia, although no one method is proven to be clinically superior, and all involve asking patients a series of questions and having them perform certain tasks. Most studies utilize the ADAS-Cog, a 70 point screening survey that measures attention, memory, orientation, language, and praxis (the ability to learn new information). Many studies also employ the CBIS, a clinical global assessment which involves both physician and caregiver impression of change and can assess more clinically relevant parameters of improvement or decline.

The US Preventive Services Task Force states that evidence is inconclusive to recommend for or against routine dementia screening. No screening method has been proven to change outcome considerably or to be entirely reliable. The harms of screening, which cannot be measured, include inducing depression/anxiety in a patient or family told they have dementia, labeling people with dementia in a way that can prevent them from obtaining long-term care insurance or even entry into retirement communities, and subjecting them to testing and treatments that could be deleterious. But, according to the USPTSF, "The most important problem with the evidence for screening for dementia is the uncertainty about the effectiveness of treatment for people whose disease would be detected by screening."[1]

Various drugs do exist to treat symptoms in dementia. None cure or slow the progress of the disease, but, like acetaminophen for arthritis or dopamine for Parkinson's, they can ameliorate symptoms. According to the Alzheimer's Association: "At this

---

[1] http://www.uspreventiveservicestaskforce.org/uspstf/uspsdeme.htm.

time, there is no treatment to cure, delay or stop the progression of Alzheimer's disease. FDA-approved drugs temporarily slow worsening of symptoms for about 6 to 12 months, on average, for about half of the individuals who take them."[2]

Two basic classes of drug treatment exist. Cholinesterase Inhibitors are the most common and best studied dementia drugs, and four of these are available, the most well-known of which is Donepezil (Aricept™). They can cause nausea, vomiting, weight loss, and diarrhea. The NMDA Antagonist Memantine (Namenda™) also has been widely used, although less studied, and it is recommended in later stages of dementia. Some patients do improve rapidly with these drugs, some show no improvement, and most demonstrate a small to modest decline in disease progression for 6-12 months. No large study of these drugs has looked at outcome beyond a year. Most improvement is noted on the ADAS-Cog [3] rather than more clinically relevant measures of dementia.

A large number of studies looking at the Cholinesterase Inhibitors have demonstrated modest improvement, especially in the ADAS score, although many people drop out of the studies from side effects [4–6]. Typically with these drugs improvement occurred early in treatment and by 18–30 weeks the people taking medicine mentally declined similarly to those taking placebo [7]. If the drugs were stopped at any juncture during treatment, then patients resorted to the same ADAS scores that they would have achieved had they not taken the drug [8]. One study measured the impact of Aricept™ on the progression of Mild Cognitive Impairment or early dementia to clinically significant dementia for a period longer than a year. Donepezil did slow the progression in the first year of treatment, but by the third year of treatment there was no difference between it and the placebo [9]. Another longer observational study also explored whether Donepezil delayed progression of patients to nursing homes and did find significant improvement over several years, [10] but that study has been widely criticized and never replicated.

Memantine is a medicine unique from the Cholinesterase Inhibitors. Although marketed as a medicine most effective in advanced Alzheimer's, it is often used early in the disease, and often given in conjunction with medicines such as Donepezil to boost the benefit of treatment. Several studies have examined the impact of Memantine on ADAS and CIBC in both early and late dementia. The improvement in ADAS is even more modest than that of Donepezil, and the improvement in CIBC is negligible. There is also no evidence that combining Memantine with a Cholinesterase Inhibitor improves the modest clinical improvement [11–14].

Although any improvement with dementia drugs seems small with ADAS criteria and clinically negligible by CIBC criteria, and typically persists for no more than six months, it is important to realize that most people exhibit no measurable improvement even by those standards. A 2008 *Annals of Internal Medicine* study defined a clinically relevant change in the ADAS score to be an improvement of 4 points or better, something not achieved by most of the prior studies that showed a positive result with drug treatment. Any change in CIBC was considered clinically significant. The authors conclude: "Treatment of dementia with Cholinesterase

---

[2] www.alz.org.

Inhibitors and Memantine can result in statistically significant but clinically marginal improvement in measures of cognition and global assessment of dementia." [15] In this analysis, approximately 110–300/1,000 patients did improve greater than four points when compared to placebo, whereas the change in CIBC was too inconsistent to interpret. Overall there were more responders on the 10 mg Aricept™ dose than the 5 mg dose with ADAS criteria, but in CIBC there was not a consistent dose response [16]. Another large meta-analysis found that 92/1,000 demented patients had a clinically significant improvement compared to placebo as defined by ADAS>4 or a meaningful CIBC change in the right direction [17]. There have been no definitive studies of the higher 23 mg dose of Donepezil that demonstrates significant improvement, especially in CIBC scores [18].

In many of the studies cited, patients taking Cholinesterase Inhibitors experienced a large number of side effects compared to placebo, typically nausea, vomiting, and diarrhea. Approximately 100/1,000 patients taking Cholinesterase Inhibitors withdrew from the studies due to side effects when compared to the placebo group. For the 23 mg dose of Donepezil there was an extremely marked increase in side-effect induced withdrawals even compared to the 10 mg dose.[3] The meta-analysis cited above found a drop-out rate in people taking active drug of 70/1,000 compared to placebo due to side effects. More serious side effects can occur as well. One study found that in patients who took Cholinesterase Inhibitors, there were 13/1,000 episodes of syncope, 2.5/1,000 hospitalizations for slow heart rate, 1.4/1,000 placements of pacemaker due to slow heart rate, and 2.6/1,000 hip fractures in excess of those who took placebo [19]. It is still unclear if more side effect information will emerge as these studies are extended to longer durations of time.

Of note, in most of the dementia drug studies there was a substantial placebo effect. The Annals study demonstrated that an average of 300/1,000 placebo-taking participants had a clinically significant ADAS response, and there were 100–300/1,000 of placebo-taking participants who exhibited a clinically significant CBIC response. While more of the drug-taking subjects had a response than the placebo-taking subjects, both numbers were very high. Therefore, for an individual patient or family assessing whether a certain dementia drug has been effective, a large number of positive responders will be exhibiting the placebo effect.

References

1. iCasey, D., et al. (2010). Drugs for Alzheimer's disease: Are they effective? *Pharmacy and Therapeutics, 35*(4), 208–211.
2. Mark-Clarfield, A. (2003). The decreasing prevalence of reversible dementias an updated meta-analysis. *Archives of Internal Medicine, 163*(18), 2219–2229.
3. Casey, D., et al. (2010). Drugs for Alzheimer's disease: Are they effective? *Pharmacy and Therapeutics, 35*(4), 208–211.
4. Birks, J. (2006). Cholinesterase Inhibitors for Alzheimer's disease. *Cochrane Database Systematic Review* (1).

---

[3] http://www.ahrp.org/cms/content/view/813/56.

5. Kavirajan, H., & Schneider, L. (2007). Efficacy and adverse effects of cholinesterase inhibitors and memantine in vascular dementia: a meta-analysis of randomised controlled trials. *The Lancet Neurology, 6*(9), 782–792.

6. Winblad, B., et al. (2001). A 1-year, randomized, placebo-controlled study of donepezil in patients with mild to moderate AD. *Neurology, 57*, 489–495.

7. Howard, R., et al. (2012). Donepezil and memantine for moderate severe Alzheimer's disease. *New England Journal of Medicine, 366*, 893–903.

8. Rainer, M., et al. (2001). Cognitive relapse after discontinuation of drug therapy in Alzheimer's disease: Cholinesterase inhibitors versus nootropics. *Journal of Neural Transmission, 108*(11), 1327–1333.

9. Petersen, R. C. (2005). Vitamin E and donepezil for the treatment of mild cognitive impairment. *New England Journal of Medicine, 353*(23), 2379–2388.

10. Geldmacher, D. S., et al. (2003). Donepezil is associated with delayed nursing home placement in patients with Alzheimer's disease. *Journal of American Geriatrics Society, 51*(7), 937–944.

11. Schneider, L., et al. (2011). Lack of evidence for the efficacy of memantine in mild Alzheimer disease. *Archives of Neurology, 68*(8), 991–998.

12. Areosa, S. A. et al. (2005). Memantine for dementia. *Cochrane Database Systematic Review* (3).

13. Howard, R., et al. (2012). Donepezil and memantine for moderate severe Alzheimer's disease. *New England Journal of Medicine, 366*, 893–903.

14. Searing L (2014) *A daily dose of vitamin e may slow early Alzheimer's disease," the Washington post*. January 4, 2014, p. E3. This study had an arm that looked at Memantine and showed no clinical improvement; Vitamin E did better in regard to ADL improvement.

15. Raina, P., et al. (2008). Effectiveness of cholinesterase inhibitors and memantine for treating dementia: Evidence review for a clinical practice guideline. *Annals of Internal Medicine, 148*(5), 379–397.

16. Qaseem, A., et al. (2008). Current pharmacologic treatment of dementia: A clinical practice guideline from the American college of physicians and the American academy of family physicians. *Annals of Internal Medicine, 148*(5), 370–378.

17. Lanctot, K., et al. (2003). Efficacy and safety of cholinesterase inhibitors in Alzheimer's disease: A meta-analysis. *Canadian Medical Association Journal, 169*(6), 557–564.

18. Schwartz, L. (2012). How the FDA forgot the evidence: the case of donepezil 23mg. *British Medical Journal, 344*, e1086.

19. Gill, S., et al. (2009). Syncope and its consequences in patients with dementia receiving cholinesterase inhibitors. *Archives of Internal Medicine, 169*(86), 7–73.

Chapter 19
Osteoporosis: Bone Density Testing and Drug Treatment

Mrs. L came in for her annual exam. She was a healthy woman of approximately 60 years who had been seeing another doctor until recently. She scripted the visit, essentially telling me what she wanted. This included an EKG, specific blood tests, a thorough exam, and a few radiologic tests. She needed a mammogram, and it was time also for her bone density test.

I asked her when she last had a bone density test, and she told me that it was 2 years ago. Her insurance would only pay for her to have the test every 2 years, although she would prefer to have it annually. I asked her what the results had been.

"Osteopenia," she said. "Almost osteoporosis. Right on the verge. They tried me on the weekly pills a few years ago when my bones started getting thinner, but those really bothered my indigestion. So then they tried me on the every month pills, which were a lot more money, but I just didn't feel right on them. Plus, all the stuff you read about them, and what they can do to you, even cause you to break your bones, I'm not sure I would take them anyway."

I asked her a few more questions. Had she ever broken a bone in her adult life? Did she have a strong family history of breaking bones? Did she fall often? She answered no to all of those. In fact, she exercised vigorously, and had no significant limitations. I wondered why she wanted another bone density test if she felt well, had a very low risk of fracture, and would not take the medicines even if the test was abnormal.

"They have new medicines that can give you once a year, by shots," she told me. "A few of my friends get those. It may not be as bad as the pills. I suppose I could take that if my bones are getting thinner. The way I see it, there is no harm getting the test and just seeing where I am."

We discussed at what point we would treat her for bone loss even if the test showed a worsening of her osteopenia. We also talked about what she would want to achieve by having the test and by treating bone loss with medicine if the test was not normal. She told me that the goal would be to improve her bone density.

"I think that the goal of treatment should be to reduce your chance of getting a fracture," I said to her. "In my opinion your risk of fracture is very low even if the

© Springer International Publishing Switzerland 2015
E. Rifkin, A. Lazris, *Interpreting Health Benefits and Risks*,
DOI 10.1007/978-3-319-11544-3_19

bone density test shows some bone loss." I then talked to her about the efficacy of bisphosphonates in reducing fracture risk. "On top of that, there is some evidence that after 5 years of medicine use you may increase your risk of fracture even if your bone density improves, as well as possibly exposing yourself to some of the side effects you experienced with the pills," I told her. "So you have to see if this is the time in your life you would want to take these medicines, since you may not be able to take them for long."

She paused and seemed perplexed. She studied the numbers: her risk of fracture, how much that risk would be improved by taking one of the osteoporosis drugs, and the risk of her getting a fracture by being on those drugs too long. She told me to set up her mammogram for now. She would think about the bone density test a little more and decide next year; there seemed to be no rush.

A. Key Questions

- Is the patient at high risk for hip fracture? How does that risk change with aging?
- What is a patient's risk of spine fracture (compression fracture), and what are the symptoms of such fractures?
- With bisphosphonates such as Alendronate (Fosamax™), what is the reduction in hip fracture rate? What is the reduction in compression fracture?
- Are there risks of taking bisphosphonates?
- If a patient agrees to take medicine for osteoporosis, how long should the patient be treated? Is there a ceiling after which treatment is ineffective or even harmful?
- If the bone density test demonstrates clinically significant bone loss, would the patient be willing to take bisphosphonates or Forteo™, the only two available treatments approved for bone loss?
- If the patient has a normal bone density screening, and would want drug treatment if the screening worsened to the point of showing osteoporosis, when should they be screened again?
- Given that bisphosphonates have a very narrow window during which they will potentially help reduce fracture risk, typically 3–5 years, is this the optimal time to take these drugs if the bone density test is abnormal?

B. Risks and Benefits

- Osteoporosis becomes more common as people age. 100/1,000 women over age 60 have osteoporosis, while it affects 400/1,000 women over age 80. It has not been determined what the rate of hip fracture is in people based on their level of bone density.

- The death and complication rate of hip fracture is high in the elderly. 200–300/1,000 people who sustain such a fracture die within a year, and many are left physically impaired.
- Compression fractures of the spine can occur spontaneously, and are felt to be more common in those with osteoporosis, although it is not known how much more common. Overall 250–400/1,000 women develop some degree of compression fracture in their life, although many of these present without symptoms or any disability.
- **With bisphosphonates, there is felt to be a 1–2/1,000 reduction of hip fracture among those treated per year for the first 3 years of treatment; data beyond that point is more specious. In high risk groups, the hip fracture reduction is closer to 10/1,000 (Fig. 19.1).**
- Bisphosphonates reduce compression fractures by 20–60/1,000, although no data exists as to how frequently they can reduce painful or debilitating spine fractures, which comprise a minority of all such fractures.
- **Bisphosphonates cause a number of side effects that are difficult to quantify; these include acid reflux, nausea, and bone pain. The most serious side effect is fracture of the femur with minimal trauma, something that occurs more frequently after prolonged treatment. It is estimated that 20/1,000 people who take bisphosphonates beyond five years are vulnerable to femur fracture (Fig. 19.2).**
- Because of the reduced efficacy after 3 years, and the increased danger after 5 years, it is felt that bisphosphonates should be discontinued after a 3–5-year window of use. It is unclear if they can be effectively and safely started again at some future juncture.
- The rate of optimal bone density testing is not known. It takes 15 years for 100/1,000 people with mildly abnormal scans to progress to osteoporosis, and a year for 100/1,000 people with borderline scans to progress. Therefore, frequency of scans can be guided by both risk factors and by the results of previous scans.

BRCTs:
Osteoporosis: Bone Density Testing and Drug Treatment

Prevention of Hip Fractures with Bisphosphonate Treatment

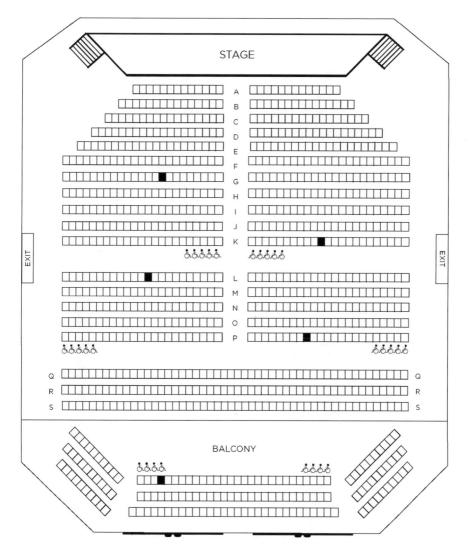

Fig. 19.1 Prevention of Hip Fractures with Bisphosphonate Treatment. Out of 1,000 women in a theater who use bisphosphonates to treat osteoporosis, 1–2 low risk people and up to 10 high risk people, average represented by blackened seats, will prevent a hip fracture compared to 1,000 people who take placebo. This benefit declines after 3 years

Risks Associated with Bisphosphonates

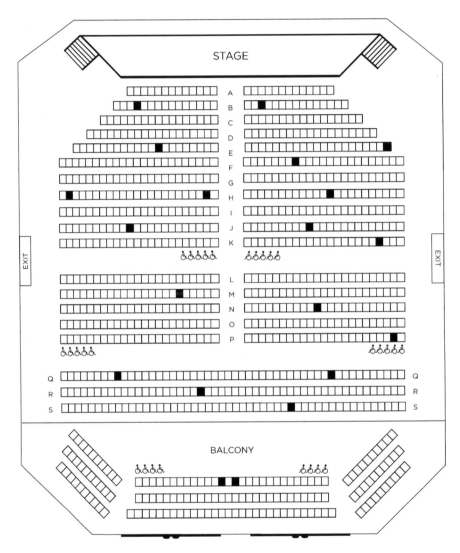

Fig. 19.2 Risks Associated with Bisphosphonates. Out of 1,000 women in a theater who use bisphosphonates for over 5 years, approximately 20 more of them, represented by blackened seats, will sustain a low-impact femur fracture than 1,000 similar women who take placebo

C. Discussion

Fractures become more common and debilitating as people age. It is estimated that 300,000 people over the age of 65 fracture a hip every year. Of those, 200–300/1,000 will die within a year of the fracture, and many of the survivors become functionally impaired.[1] Hip fractures typically lead to surgical intervention during hospitalization, followed by a prolonged stay in a rehabilitation facility, and subsequently to a decreased ability to walk and even maintain independence. Pain, blood loss, infection, mental status changes, and impaired gait are all common ramifications of hip fractures. Compression fractures of the spine afflict 250/1,000 post-menopausal women and 400/1,000 of women over the age of 80. Although many spine fractures are asymptomatic, some produce severe back pain and disability [1].

Falls contribute to hip fractures, although many compression fractures can occur even in the absence of trauma. Since falling becomes common as people age, the elderly are more vulnerable to these types of fractures. In addition, with age comes a decrease in bone density and subsequent fragility of bones. At its earlier stage this process is labeled osteopenia, and as it advances it progresses to osteoporosis, it increases a person's susceptibility to fracture. According to the International Osteoporosis Foundation, osteoporosis affects 200 million people worldwide, leading to nine million fractures annually. 100/1,000 women age 60 have osteoporosis, 200/1,000 at age 70, and 400/1,000 at age 80.[2] Many factors contribute to the development of osteoporosis including family history, age, smoking and alcohol use, inactivity, thin stature, and certain drugs such as steroids and GERD drugs called proton pump inhibitors.

Most clinical practice guidelines suggest that all women over age 65 have bone density testing, and typically insurance will pay for it as often as annually. The bone densitometry radiologic test is harmless and inexpensive. The US Preventive Services Task Force recommends bone density screening for women between the ages of 65 and 85, citing no or limited evidence to screen people outside of that age group. Screening is most effective in older women, those with more severe osteoporosis, and those with prior fractures as an adult. USPSTF recommendations do state that there is no evidence as to how often women should be screened.[3]

Why screen? The goal of bone density testing ultimately is to prevent fractures. The test can measure the density of certain bones, especially bones more prone to fracture, such as the hip and the spine. The results are relayed as a T score. The lower the T score, the more brittle the bones, and theoretically the more likely such bones are to be fractured. T scores of −1 to −2.5 are considered in the range of osteopenia. T scores of −2.5 or lower put a patient in the range of osteoporosis, which increases the risk of fracture and thus may warrant treatment.

---

[1] http://www.aarp.org/health/conditions-treatments/info-10-2011/hip-fractures-survival.html.

[2] http://www.iofbonehealth.org/facts-statistics.

[3] http://www.uspreventiveservicestaskforce.org/uspstf/uspsoste.htm.

Screening for low bone density only makes sense if an abnormal result can be treated in a way that prevents fracture and has an acceptable side effect profile. The most commonly employed medicines to treat low bone density are bisphosphonates, a class of drugs that block bone breakdown. Alendronate, or Fosamax™, is the best studied and most widely used of these, although newer annual IV forms have also become popular lately. Bisphosphonates have numerous side effects including increased acid reflux, abdominal pain, and less commonly osteonecrosis of the jaw and even spontaneous fractures of the leg.

There is evidence that bisphosphonates do improve T scores, and many studies cite a 55 % reduction in hip fracture among post-menopausal women who take Alendronate [2]. The reduction in spine fractures is even more impressive. But what is the absolute risk reduction from taking bisphosphonates? In one large Alendronate trial in a high risk group of women with an average age of 68 and an average T score −2.5, the 56 % hip fracture reduction in people who took Alendronate for 4 years conferred an absolute benefit of 2 fewer hip fractures for every 1,000 high risk women who take the drug for a year compared to those who take placebo [3].

The USPSTF recommendation to screen people over 65 relies on data showing that treatment of abnormal bone density is effective at preventing hip fractures. According to the USPSTF, the number of hip fractures prevented per year among 1,000 women screened and treated is 0.05 for women age 55-9, 0.1 for women 60–4, 0.27 for women age 65–9, and 1.4 for women age 75–9 [4]. A more recent Cochrane review stratified women into high risk (documented osteoporosis or a history of spine fracture) and low risk women (non-osteoporotic T score and no history of spine fracture). People were treated for a year or longer with bisphosphonates. In all, 10 hip fractures in high risk women were prevented for every 1,000 treated, while 0 hip fractures in low risk women were prevented [5].

The reduction of spine fractures in most analyses is more impressive than that of hip fracture with bisphosphonate users. Cochrane states that in high risk women, 60 spine fractures were prevented for every 1,000 women treated. In the lower risk group of women, 20 spine fractures were prevented. But spine fractures are not easy to quantify, because many osteoporosis studies ascertain the presence of a spine fracture only by x-ray evidence, even if the fracture is so clinically trivial that it causes the woman no pain [6]. Thus many of these women may not have had clinically significant fractures.

As to how often women should be screened, a normal bone density study usually portends a good prognosis. In post-menopausal women, less than 100/1,000 progressed to osteoporosis in 15 years in those with mild osteopenia; less than 100/1,000 progressed in 5 years in those with moderate osteopenia; and less than 100/1,000 progressed in 1 year in those with severe osteopenia [7]. Therefore, for those women who do seek screening and are normal to mildly osteopenic, after 15 years, less than 100 out of 1,000 patients will have progressed to a higher risk category.

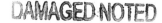
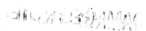

The side effects of bisphosphonates are difficult to quantify. Most studies suggest that people who take these medicines can have adverse symptoms and, more rarely, harmful effects. These include nausea, heartburn, abdominal pain, muscle and joint pain, and more seriously osteonecrosis of the jaw and gastric damage. Recently, there has been concern about one side effect that becomes more prevalent the longer women take these drugs: fracture of the femur bone in the legs induced by minimal trauma. It is felt that long-term bisphosphonate use triggers over-suppression of bone turnover, causing bones to be more fragile despite improved bone density. One recent study estimates that 20/1,000 women may be vulnerable to this serious side effect if they take the medicine for a prolonged period [8, 9]. In addition, newer studies also show that the efficacy of bisphosphonates seems to extinguish after 3–5 years, and there is no fracture risk reduction beyond that very brief window of use.[4]

Several other treatments exist for osteoporosis. Estrogens such as Premarin™ previously were a standard treatment for osteoporosis, but mortality data and limited efficacy evidence have curtailed their use in that capacity. An anti-estrogen Reloxifine, also called Evista™, has no effect on hip fracture and a modest effect on spine fracture, while it can increase the rate of deep vein thrombosis, a potentially lethal side effect.[5] Nasal Calcitonin™, which has had limited use in treating the pain of compression fractures, has been found to lack efficacy in the treatment of osteoporosis or fracture prevention, while also causing a statistical increase in cancer, leading the FDA to remove it from approved osteoporosis drugs this year.[6] Teripartide (Forteo™), a Parathyroid Hormone Derivative that helps to build bones, has an impressive impact on vertebral fractures, and by one study can prevent 30 hip fractures for every 1,000 high risk women who use it, but it has limited long-term safety data, has potential serious side effects, and is an expensive short-term medicine that has to be self-injected daily.[7] Overall, bisphosphonates continue to be the most widely used medicines for osteoporosis, and thus are what most women would take to treat an abnormal bone density test.

---

[4] http://well.blogs.nytimes.com/2012/05/09/new-cautions-about-long-term-use-of-bone-drugs.

[5] http://www.cadth.ca/en/products/health-technology-assessment/publication/502.

[6] http://www.healio.com/endocrinology/bone-mineral-metabolism/news/online/%7B5413eebd-9b1f-4ada-bd90-5bea9ef25476%7D/fda-to-review-potential-cancer-risk-associated-with-calcitonin-salmon.

[7] http://ccjm.org/content/70/7/585.full.pdf.

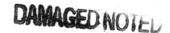

References

1. Old, J., & Calvert, M. (2004). Vertebral compression fractures in the elderly. *American Family Physician, 69*(1), 111–16.
2. Iwamoto, J., et al. (2008). Hip fracture protection by alendronate treatment in postmenopausal women with osteoporosis: A review of the literature. *Clinical Interventions in Aging, 3*(3), 483–9.
3. Abramson, *Overdosed America* (p 213)
4. Nelson, H. D., et al. (2002). Screening for postmenopausal osteoporosis: A review of the evidence for the U.S. preventive services task force. *Annals of Internal Medicine, 137*, 529–41.
5. Wells, G. A., et al. (2008). Alendronate for the primary and secondary prevention of osteoporotic fractures in postmenopausal women. *Cochrane Database of Systematic Reviews* 2008, Issue 1. Art. No.: CD001155. DOI: 10.1002/14651858.CD001155.pub2; Cochrane Database of Systematic Reviews, "Alendronate for preventing fractures caused by osteoporosis in postmenopausal women", First published: January 23, 2008
6. Hadler, *Rethinking aging* (p 121)
7. Gourlay, M. L., et al. (2012). Bone density testing intervals and transition to osteoporosis in older women. *New England Journal of Medicine, 366*, 225–32.
8. LaRocca Vieira, R., et al. (2012). Frequency of incomplete atypical femoral fractures in asymptomatic patients on long-term bisphosphonate therapy. *American Journal of Roentgenology, 198*(5), 1144–51.
9. Shneider, J. P. (2009). Bisphosphonates and low-impact femoral fractures: current evidence on alendronate-fracture risk. *Geriatrics, 64*(1), 18–23.

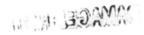

Chapter 20
Osteoporosis: Calcium and Vitamin D

Mrs. R was concerned about her bones. Her mother had fractures at an old age, and she was once told she had some thinning of the bones. She took calcium regularly and fairly high doses of Vitamin D. She had a Vitamin D level checked annually and the last one was in the 40's. She wondered if she should take more so she could attain a higher level. Some of her friends told her that the level should be in the 50's, and she read about the importance of Vitamin D in one of her medical newsletters.

She was in her 70's and was fairly active. She had not broken any bones. Her balance had deteriorated over the years, and now she used a cane at times, especially when traversing uneven outdoor surfaces. She had been on an osteoporosis drug Boniva™ (a bisphosphonate) in the past but could not tolerate it. She typically liked to treat illness more naturally than with using medicines.

"I take 1,200 mg of calcium and over 2,000u of Vitamin D3," she told me. "Is that enough?"

We discussed the pros and cons of calcium supplementation. She had read that there was some controversy about it, but she knew that it was good for the bones, and that without it her bones could become fragile and ultimately break. We discussed her dietary sources of calcium, including milk and cereal. I talked about the relationship between ingested calcium and bone health, and showed her a BRCT. She had a difficult time accepting that calcium may not be necessary to keep her bones strong.

In regard to Vitamin D, she believed that her level should be higher, even after we discussed the limits of current data. We talked about the potential benefits of Vitamin D supplements to her health, and the potential risks of taking too much D. She told me that she read that Vitamin D helped more than just the bones, and could actually prevent heart attacks and certain cancers. We talked about that as well. After our conversation, she decided to decrease her calcium dose and to maintain her current dose of Vitamin D, requesting that I check another D level next year.

© Springer International Publishing Switzerland 2015
E. Rifkin, A. Lazris, *Interpreting Health Benefits and Risks*,
DOI 10.1007/978-3-319-11544-3_20

A. Key Questions

- Does the patient obtain enough calcium in his/her diet?
- Does the patient get enough Vitamin D through dietary sources and sun expo-sure? What is the Vitamin D level?
- If the patient has osteoporosis, would there be any benefit in taking calcium with regard to reducing fracture risk?
- Are there any dangers of taking calcium supplementation?
- Would there be any benefit of taking Vitamin D?
- How much Vitamin D should a patient take, and how often should doctors monitor the levels? Is there a danger of taking too much Vitamin D?

B. Risks and Benefits

- Calcium is very common in food while Vitamin D is not. To achieve adequate daily consumption, most people do not have to take calcium supplementation, but typically they do have to take Vitamin D.
- Vitamin D levels in the blood can determine if someone is deficient. Calcium levels in the blood are less helpful.
- A small study of institutionalized elderly showed a 7/1,000 reduction in hip frac-ture rate with supplementation of calcium with Vitamin D compared to placebo. In a study of calcium supplementation alone without Vitamin D, there was a 9/1,000 *increase* in hip fracture rate compared to placebo.
- Calcium does have several side effects such as constipation, increase rate of kidney stones, and gas. Some studies suggest that calcium supplementation increases the risk of vascular events (heart attack, stroke, cardiac bypass) by 6/1,000 compared to those not taking supplementation.
- **Vitamin D may decrease the hip fracture rate by 0–4/1,000 compared to placebo, but it is unclear which people benefit most from supplementation (Fig. 20.1).**
- **Vitamin D supplementation may reduce the risk of falling by 95/1,000 com-pared to placebo in those who achieve fairly high levels and who are prone to falls (Fig. 20.2).**
- **No studies of calcium supplementation show a definitive decrease in frac-ture rate, and most positive studies use a combination of Calcium and D (Fig. 20.3).**
- Vitamin D is a fat soluble vitamin that can reach toxic levels if taken in excess. Studies have demonstrated a small increased risk of death with very high and low levels. In those who achieve very high levels of Vitamin D by taking mega-supplementation, there is a 31/1,000 *increased* rate of hip fracture and a 324/1,000 *increased* risk of falls.

BRCTs:
Osteoporosis: Calcium and Vitamin D

Vitamin D Averting Hip Fractures

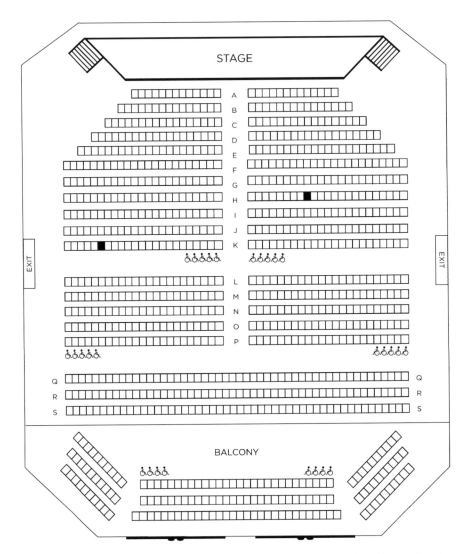

Fig. 20.1 Vitamin D Averting Hip Fractures. Out of 1,000 women sitting in a theater who take Vitamin D regularly, 0–4 of them will avert a hip fracture, average represented by blackened seats, over a variable number of years compared to 1,000 women who take placebo

Vitamin D and Fall Prevention

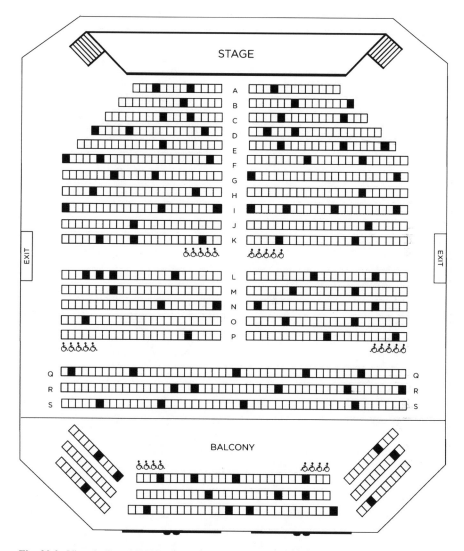

Fig. 20.2 Vitamin D and Fall Prevention. Out of 1,000 women in a theater who take Vitamin D regularly and achieve a fairly high Vitamin D level in their blood, 95, represented by blackened seats, will avoid falling compared to 1,000 women who take placebo

Calcium Preventing Hip Fractures

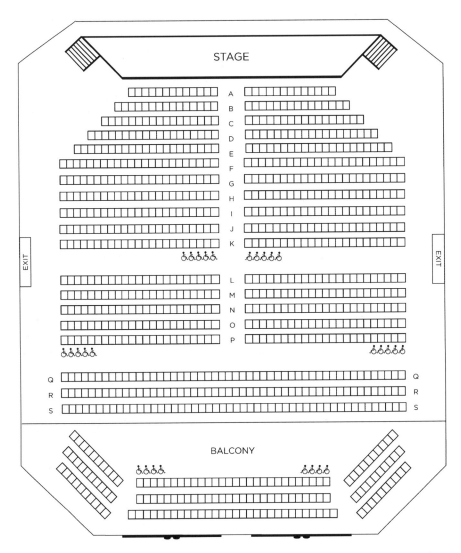

Fig. 20.3 Calcium Preventing Hip Fractures. Out of 1,000 women in a theater who take calcium supplementation without Vitamin D, no study has demonstrated any reduction of hip fracture rate, as represented by the absence of blackened seats. Some studies, in fact, show a slightly higher hip fracture rate

C. Discussion

As previously discussed, osteoporosis impacts a large number of women as they age, making them more prone to debilitating fractures, especially of the hip and spine. Those patients prone to falls are more vulnerable to sustaining hip fractures. We talked about the implications of bone density screening and drug treatment of osteoporosis in a prior chapter. It is also important to note that deficiencies of calcium and Vitamin D can precipitate bone loss and consequent fracture. Calcium is needed to build bones and maintain their strength, while Vitamin D helps with calcium absorption into the body and bones. Currently more than half of women in the country take calcium and Vitamin D supplements to maintain their bone health. Many organizations, such as the International Osteoporosis Foundation, recommend calcium and Vitamin D supplementation in older women in an effort to improve bone strength and avert osteoporosis.[1] In addition to helping bone density, Vitamin D is also believed to reduce the rate of falls, another major contributor to fracture risk.

Both calcium and Vitamin D can be obtained naturally. Calcium is fairly ubiquitous in the American diet and can be found in dairy products, fish, cabbage, and fortified breads/cereals/juices. Many medical groups, such as the NIH, recommend that older women consume 1,200 mg of calcium a day, an amount fairly easy to achieve with a balanced diet. Vitamin D is less available in food; fortified dairy contains approximately 10 % of daily D per serving, and salmon, which has the highest concentration of Vitamin D, contains about half of the daily requirement. Sun exposure is an excellent source of D, but patients must be in direct sunlight for 5–30 min with skin exposed and without sunscreen to have sufficient absorption. Currently older people are recommended to consume at least 800iu of Vitamin D a day.[2]

Vitamin D can be measured in the blood, and the upper and lower limits of therapeutic levels have been defined. Because D is a fat soluble Vitamin, excess use of it can lead to toxic levels, as it is not flushed out of the body like most water soluble vitamins. While calcium too can be measured in the blood, its levels do not correlate to bone concentrations. Excess calcium levels can precipitate serious medical complications including kidney stones and cardiac arrhythmias. Calcium supplementation can cause gas and constipation, especially in the elderly. The goals of supplementing calcium and Vitamin D are both to improve bone density and, more significantly, to prevent fractures.

Calcium: Several studies have evaluated the efficacy of calcium supplementation in its impact on bone density and fracture risk. Most studies provide inconclusive results. Subsequently, the US Preventive Services Task Force gives no recommendation as to whether women with or without osteoporosis should supplement their diet with calcium.[3] A review of available studies concluded the following: "No

---

[1] http://www.iofbonehealth.org/facts-statistics.

[2] http://ods.od.nih.gov/factsheets/Calcium-HealthProfessional/.

[3] http://www.uspreventiveservicestaskforce.org/uspstf/uspsvitd.htm.

single study has credibly demonstrated a reduction in vertebral, non-vertebral, or hip fracture incidence with calcium supplementation. Evidence that calcium supplementation reduces the risk of vertebral, non-vertebral, or hip fracture is derived from meta-analyses of these problematic trials. But even the meta-analyses provide inconsistent information, and several suggest that hip fracture rates are increased in the calcium-supplemented groups." [1]

In the Women's Health Initiative, a long-term trial of 36,000 post-menopausal women under the age of 80, there was no statistically significant difference in fracture rate between women who took calcium/Vitamin D supplementation and those who did not. Total data suggests a trend toward improvement, with two fewer hip fractures per 1,000 people who took calcium with vitamin D, and one fewer spine fractures per 1,000 women who took calcium with Vitamin D [2].

A large meta-analysis did suggest a reduction of fracture rate with calcium and D supplementation, but critics of the study suggested that it used data that was not reliable. Much of the benefit was seen in institutionalized elderly people with baseline low calcium/d intake, as well as in people who took large amounts of Vitamin D. The calcium and vitamin D combination group did have approximately 7/1,000 fewer fractures overall [3, 4]. It is important to realize that in all of these studies of calcium supplementation, treatment subjects also received Vitamin D, something that may have skewed the results. In fact, an analysis of calcium supplementation without Vitamin D demonstrated just the opposite results of the Calcium/D studies, with 9/1,000 *more* hip fractures in the calcium group than those who took placebo [5].

Recently there has been speculation that calcium supplementation may increase the risk of heart attacks, something that has generated a great deal of controversy. A large study reexamining the Women's Health Initiative data found that women not previously taking calcium had an increased rate of vascular disease once they took a calcium/Vitamin D supplement regularly over the duration of the study. With supplementation there was a 4/1,000 increase in heart attacks, 3/1,000 increase in stroke, and 6/1,000 increase in the combined endpoint of heart attack, revascularization, and cardiac death. There was no significant change in overall death [6]. An early randomized trial by the same author found similar results [7]. A more recent NIH study, with a different design, found an increase in coronary artery disease in men but not women [8]. Clearly more study is required, but calcium given to those who have not taken it seems to confer some cardiac risk.

Vitamin D: Several studies have shown beneficial effects of Vitamin D supplementation in the prevention of fracture, most notably among women with baseline low Vitamin D levels. A pooled study of 31,000 women over the age of 65 found that women who took Vitamin D supplements had 4/1,000 fewer hip fractures than did women on placebo. The results only reached statistical significance at higher Vitamin D doses, and there was great variability between studies [9]. A large study conducted for the US Preventive Services Task Force highlights some of the confusion regarding Vitamin D and fracture risk. The study did show a mild improvement with Vitamin D use concomitant with calcium, but it was unclear how pre-study D levels and overall D dose impacted results [10]. Most recently a meta-analysis looked at Vitamin D and its impact on bone density and found disparate results, [11] although there is not necessarily a correlation between bone density and fracture risk.

One reason Vitamin D may improve fracture risk is that it seems to have an impact in reducing falls among the elderly. Currently the USPSTF recommends the use of Vitamin D supplementation in community dwelling elderly people who are at high risk for falls.[4] A large meta-analysis of seven studies involving 1,900 elderly people over 65 who took moderate doses of Vitamin D (700–1,000 units) for 1–3 years found a significant decrease in fall rate among those taking Vitamin D. The treated group had an absolute fall reduction of 95/1,000 people treated compared to placebo. There was no significant fall reduction among those who took lower doses and among those who did not achieve a relatively high blood level of D (60) [12].

Of note, because Vitamin D is a fat soluble vitamin, it is possible to achieve toxic levels when doses are too high. In addition, high doses may actually reduce some of the vitamin's benefits on outcome. A large observational study looking at total mortality in 250,000 people found that those with low and high Vitamin D levels had an increase in death rate compared to those whose range was normal [13]. In a placebo-controlled trial of 2,250 elderly women at high risk of falling, followed for 3-5 years, women receiving very high D doses sustained 31/1,000 excess fractures and 324/1,000 excess falls compared to those receiving placebo [14]. At present, the optimal dose of Vitamin D to prevent falls and fractures has not been ascertained.

References

1. Seeman, E. (2010). Evidence that calcium supplements reduce fracture risk is lacking. *Clinical Journal of American Society of Nephrology, 2010*(5), S3–S11.
2. Jackson, R. D., et al. (2006). Calcium plus vitamin D supplementation and the risk of fractures. *New England Journal of Medicine, 354*(7), 669–683.
3. Tang, B. M., et al. (2007). Use of calcium or calcium in combination with vitamin D supplementation to prevent fractures and bone loss in people aged 50 years and older: A meta-analysis. *Lancet, 370,* 657–666.
4. Freychuss, B., et al. (2007). Calcium and vitamin D for prevention of osteoporotic fractures. *Lancet, 2007*(370), 2098–2099.
5. Reid, I. R., & Bolland, M. J. (2008). Effect of calcium supplementation on hip fractures. *Osteoporosis International, 2008*(19), 1119–1123.
6. Bolland, M. J., et al. (2011). Calcium supplements with or without vitamin D and risk of cardiovascular events: Reanalysis of the women's health initiative. *British Medical Journal, 342,* d2040.
7. Bolland, M. J., et al. (2008). Vascular events in healthy older women receiving calcium supplementation. *British Medical Journal, 336,* 262–266.
8. Xiao, Q., et al. (2013). Dietary and supplemental calcium intake and cardiovascular disease mortality the national institutes of health – AARP Diet and Health Study. *Journal of American Medical Association Internal Medicine, 173*(8), 639–646.

---

[4] http://www.uspreventiveservicestaskforce.org/uspstf/uspsfalls.htm.

 9. Bischoff-Ferrari, H. A., et al. (2012). A pooled analysis of vitamin d dose requirements for fracture prevention. *New England Journal of Medicine, 367*, 40–49.
10. Chung, M., et al. (2011). Vitamin D with or without calcium supplementation for prevention of cancer and fractures: an updated meta-analysis for the U.S. preventive services task force. *Annals of Internal Medicine, 155*(12), 827–838.
11. Bolland, M. J., et al. (2014). Effect of vitamin D supplementation on bone mineral density. *Lancet, 2014*(383), 146–155.
12. Bischoff-Ferrari, H. A., et al. (2009). Fall prevention with supplemental and active forms of vitamin D: A meta-analysis of randomized controlled trials. *British Medical Journal, 339*, b3692.
13. Durup, D., et al. (2012). A reverse J-shaped association of all-cause mortality with serum 25-hydroxyvitamin D in general practice: The CopD study. *Journal of Clinical Endocrinolgy and Metabolism, 97*(8), 2644–2652.
14. Sanders, K. M., et al. (2010). Annual high-dose oral vitamin D and falls and fractures in older women: A randomized controlled trial. *Journal of American Medical Association, 303*(18), 1815–1822.

Chapter 21
Estrogen Replacement Therapy

Mrs. R came in to the office desperate. She was in her late 50's and her menstrual periods started to slow approximately 2 years ago. Now she had no bleeding, something she appreciated, but other symptoms appeared. She was having waves of hot flushes, often followed by sweats. This could occur at the most inopportune times, such as during the night, or even at work when she was making a presentation. She also felt more tired and anxious, and she was convinced that she was losing her hair. "Overall," she told me with a sigh, "I'm falling apart."

Having read the internet and talked to friends, she suspected that some of her symptoms derived from being in menopause. She was not an avid exerciser, but was told by one friend that exercise could help. She did go to the gym several times a week now, something she was happy about with regard to her overall health and a subsequent drop in weight, but the symptoms of menopause persisted. She also tried many over-the-counter remedies she found in health food stores and on the internet. Initially some seemed to help her, but their effect did not persist.

I told her that most studies show no improvement in menopausal symptoms with over-the- counter products or even most prescription medicines. In fact, placebo did just as well, and as many as half of women who took placebo had temporary relief that did not persist.

"Well," she said, "I guess I have to just deal with it. How long do you think it could last?"

I told her that the symptom duration varied but could persist for many more years. That did not make her very happy.

"What about using estrogen?" I asked. "That takes care of those symptoms in virtually everyone."

She looked at me as though I was insane. "I mean, I don't like feeling hot and losing my hair, but it's not worth dying of breast cancer to treat it."

I talked to her a bit about estrogen replacement. Since she had a uterus, she would likely want to take a combination of estrogen and another hormone, Premarin™ (progesterone), to avoid the small but real increased risk of uterine cancer in those who take estrogen alone. That would cause her to have some spotting,

© Springer International Publishing Switzerland 2015
E. Rifkin, A. Lazris, *Interpreting Health Benefits and Risks*,
DOI 10.1007/978-3-319-11544-3_21

something that likely would resolve in a few months. I then showed her data about the risks of taking estrogen, especially the risks of stroke, cancer, heart disease, and blood clot that were found in the Women's Health Initiative study. She looked at it somewhat quizzically. "That's it?" she asked. "That's hardly anyone who gets problems. Why is there so much talk about how bad it is to take estrogen?"

I then showed her the absolute numbers as to how estrogen may impact someone her age. She was astounded, almost to the point of disbelief. She had to have me repeat the numbers again.

"Then if this is all true, why is everyone telling me not to take estrogen?"

I shrugged.

She immediately asked me to write her a prescription for hormones. I did offer her the option of taking estrogen alone, which would slightly increase her absolute risk of uterine cancer but not cause her to have spotting. She chose the combination pill. Within three months, when I heard from her again, her menopausal symptoms had completely abated, and her slight spotting had disappeared. Now she wanted to know how long she could take this. She felt great.

A. Key Questions

- What are symptoms of menopause, and how can they be treated?
- How effective is estrogen in alleviating the symptoms of menopause? Are there side effects?
- Who can take estrogen alone, and who has to take a combination of estrogen and progesterone? Are there additional side effects of using the latter?
- What are the risks of hip fracture, stroke, heart disease, blood clot, and breast cancer overall in women who use estrogen?
- In women under the age of 60 who take estrogen soon after menopause, what are the long-term health effects of using hormone replacement?
- In older women over the age of 70 who start estrogen, what are the long-term health effects?

B. Risks and Benefits

- Hot flushes, sweats, and vaginal dryness are the primary symptoms of menopause. Most prescription and over-the-counter remedies do not appreciably ameliorate these.
- **Estrogen replacement improves menopausal symptoms in 900/1,000 women who use it. Most women do not have significant side effects, but that varies (Fig. 21.1).**
- Women with a uterus are at a higher risk of uterine cancer if they use estrogen. Therefore, they are usually told to use progesterone with the estrogen. This can

cause some spotting for several months after use. It is unclear what the absolute risk is of using unopposed estrogen in women with a uterus both in terms of cancer development and cancer death.

- Overall women using hormone replacement therapy have a decreased hip fracture risk of 5.5/1,000, an increased leg clot(DVT)/pulmonary embolism risk of 1/1,000, and increased non-fatal stroke risk of 1/1,000 over those who take placebo, although many of these strokes are not disabling. There is a 1/1,000 decreased breast cancer risk in estrogen users, and a 1/1,000 increased breast cancer risk in estrogen–progesterone users compared to placebo, but no change in breast cancer mortality. There is a similar decline in colon cancer risk in both groups of 1/1,000. Hormone replacement therapy seems to have no overall impact on the risk of death.
- **Young women who initiate hormones soon after menopause seem to have a reduced mortality of between 6 and 23/1,000 compared to non-estrogen users (Fig.** 21.2**).**
- Also young women who initiate hormones soon after menopause have reduced cancer mortality of 17/1,000, a decrease in cardiac events of 34/1,000 without change in cardiac mortality, and an increase in non-fatal stroke of 1–6/1,000 compared to non-users. There was no change in the risk of leg clot (DVT).
- Older women who initiate estrogen have an increase in mortality of 23/1,000 and an increased cardiac event rate of 2/1,000, with similar stroke risk to younger women.

BRCTs:
Estrogen Replacement Therapy

Effectiveness of Estrogen in Treating Menopausal Symptoms

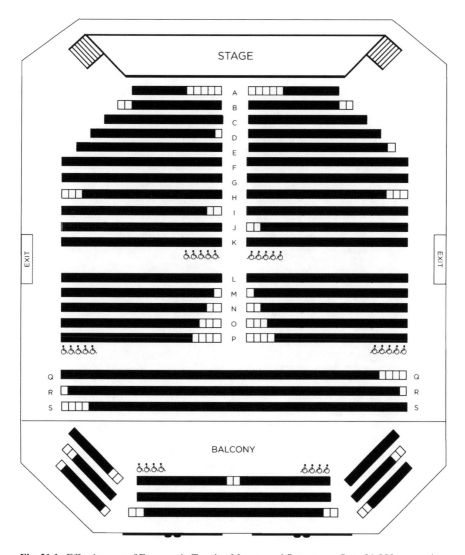

Fig. 21.1 Effectiveness of Estrogen in Treating Menopausal Symptoms. Out of 1,000 women in a theater with menopausal symptoms who take estrogen, 900 of them, represented by blacked seats, will have significant improvement in symptoms compared to 1,000 women who take a placebo

Risks of Taking Estrogen for Post-menopausal Women

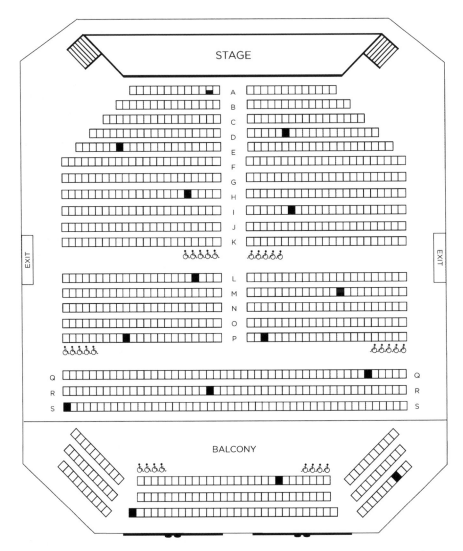

Fig. 21.2 Risks of Taking Estrogen for Post-menopausal Women. Out of 1,000 women in a theater who take estrogen soon after the onset of menopause, 6–23 of them, average represented by blackened seats, will have an overall decreased death rate compared to 1,000 women who take a placebo

C. Discussion

During menopause, women have a fairly rapid depletion of their estrogen levels, leading to various symptoms and physiological changes. Many women experience hot flushes, sweats, urinary frequency, and vaginal dryness. Often these symptoms can be debilitating and persist for years. Many over-the-counter herbal and pharmaceutical treatments exist, but their efficacy is no better than placebo. The most effective remedy for menopausal symptoms is estrogen, typical available as a synthetic formulation that can be taken daily. The vast majority of women who take estrogen after menopause (900/1,000) have complete symptom relief[1] [1]. In addition to symptoms, the onset of menopause instigates changes within a woman's body that may induce an acceleration of osteoporosis and perhaps even an increase in heart disease. For many years, it was believed that estrogen replacement would not only provide symptom relief, but also other health benefits.

One well-recognized danger of estrogen use in women with an intact uterus is an increase in the rate of uterine cancer. That risk has been documented in studies of relative risk, [2] but little is known of the absolute risk of taking unopposed estrogen, nor is there ample data to determine if estrogen use contributes to elevated cancer death or any increase in mortality. Regardless, it is considered standard of care to use another hormone, progesterone, in conjunction with estrogen in women with a uterus, thereby mitigating the risk of uterine cancer. The use of progesterone can cause post-menopausal women to have some degree of vaginal bleeding that usually extinguishes in a few months, and it is unknown if progesterone increases health risk.

More recently, primarily due to the publication of a large randomized trial of post-menopausal estrogen use called the Women's Health Initiative (WHI), the health dangers of both estrogen and estrogen combined with progesterone have been highlighted, and the use of estrogen after menopause has dramatically declined. The US Preventive Services Task Force now recommends against the use of estrogen in post-menopausal women, citing the fact that the risks of use exceed benefit.[2] But without estrogen, many women must now confront menopause without any viable treatments. Therefore, the question becomes just how risky estrogen use may be, and is that risk enough to dissuade women from using estrogen to obtain symptom relief?

For users of estrogen, the USPSTF cites an increase risk of stroke of 1.1/1,000 and dvt (clot) of the leg of 0.7/1,000 compared to placebo. There is an actually a *decreased* risk of hip fracture among users of 5.6/1,000, breast cancer of 0.8/1,000, and of death of 0.2/1,000. When estrogen is combined with progesterone there is similar reduction of hip fracture and increase rate of stroke. However, there is an increased risk of breast cancer of 0.8/1,000, of dvt of 1.3/1,000, and of pulmonary embolism of 0.9/1,000. All users of estrogen had more incontinence, and some had

---

[1] http://usatoday30.usatoday.com/news/health/medical/health/medical/womenshealth/story/2012-01-16/Hot-flash-remedies-Estrogen-may-be-the-best-answer/52604096/1.

[2] http://www.uspreventiveservicestaskforce.org/uspstf12/menohrt/menohrtart.htm.

an increased in dementia [3]. The WHI also shows a 0.7/1,000 increased risk of coronary artery disease in those who use estrogen with progesterone, although there was no increase in fatal heart attacks or cardiac death. There was a decrease in incidence of colon cancer in the study that was similar to the increase in breast cancer [4]. It is important to note that both the WHI and the USPSTF do not comment on whether estrogen increases the risk of debilitating strokes (those in which symptoms persist) or breast cancer deaths.

A critique of the WHI is that many of the women studied were far older than the typical post-menopausal woman who would be requesting hormone replacement. When only younger women are examined, the results changed fairly dramatically. A review of WHI data showed that in women between ages 50 and 59 who initiated estrogen replacement with and without progesterone, there was a *decrease* in mortality of 6.4/1,000, and a slight decrease in cardiac events compared to non-users, although the risk of non-fatal stroke remained slightly higher than non-users (by 1.3/1,000). In women who started using estrogen within ten years of menopause, there was a similar decrease in morality and cardiac events. Contrarily, older women (ages 70–79) who started estrogen had a 23/1,000 increase in mortality and 1.9/1,000 increase in cardiac events compared to non-users, and those who started estrogen use more than 20 years after menopause had a 7.2/1,000 increase in mortality. Therefore, the bulk of adverse effects of estrogen use in the WHI occurred in older women, whose large numbers in the study skewed results toward demonstrating harmful effects [5].

Several more recent studies have looked specifically at the impact of estrogen on younger women. Two pooled analyses of studies found a measurable drop in mortality in young women who take estrogen soon after menopause compared to those who do not. One study looked at 30 trials with an average follow-up of 4.5 years, and found that in women under 60 who took estrogen there was a 23/1,000 drop in mortality, 17/1,000 drop in cancer mortality, and no change in cardiac mortality [6]. Another study by the same author looked at 17 trials of younger women, mean age 55, for 14 years and found a 10/1,000 decrease in mortality among those who used estrogen compared to those who did not [7].

A randomized trial of 1,000 younger women who used estrogen or estrogen–progesterone after menopause followed for 11 years found that hormone users had a 22/1,000 decrease in mortality, 34/1,000 decrease in cardiac events, 6/1,000 increase in non-fatal strokes, and 14/1,000 increase in non-fatal breast cancer. There was no change in DVT rate [8]. The KEEPS trial is following the health impact of estrogen on young women who initiate hormonal treatment within 3 years of menopause, having found significant improvement in menopausal symptoms without any adverse health risks.[3] One recent analysis has even suggested that thousands of younger post-menopausal women die every year by being denied estrogen, especially if they do not have a uterus [9]. Without a doubt estrogen does improve symptoms of menopause for the vast majority of women who use it. As new research emerges, the harmful impact of estrogen is being questioned, especially on those women who use estrogen at the time of menopause.

---

[3] http://www.menopause.org/docs/agm/general-release.pdf?sfvrsn=0.

References

1. Barrett-Connor, E., & Stuenkel, C. (2001). Hormone replacement therapy: Risks and benefits. *International Journal of Epidemiology, 30*(3), 423–426.
2. Grady, D., et al. (1995). Hormone replacement therapy and endometrial cancer risk: A meta-analysis. *Obstetrics and Gynecology, 85*(2), 304–312.
3. Moyer, V., et al. (2012). Menopausal hormone replacement therapy for primary prevention of chronic conditions: US preventive services task force recommendation statement. *Annals of Internal Medicine, 158*, 47–54.
4. Investigators, W. H. I., et al. (2002). Risks and benefits of estrogen plus progestin in healthy postmenopausal womenprincipal results from the women's health initiative randomized controlled trial. *Journal of American Medical Association, 288*(3), 321–333.
5. Russouw, J., & Reckelhoff, J. (2007). Postmenopausal hormone therapy and risk of coronary vascular disease by age and years since menopause. *Journal of American Medical Association, 297*(13), 1465–1477.
6. Salpeter, S., et al. (2004). Mortality associate with hormone replacement therapy in younger and older women. *Journal of General Internal Medicine, 19*(7), 791–804.
7. Salpeter, S., et al. (2009). Bayesian meta-analysis of hormone therapy and mortality in younger post-menopausal women. *The American Journal of Medicine, 122*(11), 1016–1022.
8. Schierbeck, L., et al. (2012). Effect of hormone replacement therapy on cardiovascular events in recently postmenopausal women: Randomised trial. *British Medical Journal, 345*, e6409.
9. Sarrel, P., et al. (2013). The mortality toll of estrogen avoidance: an analysis of excess deaths among hysterectomized women aged 50 to 59 years. *American Journal of Public Health, 103*(9), 1583–1588.

Chapter 22
Vitamins and Supplements

Mrs. W liked taking vitamins. She was convinced that natural remedies were superior to medicines, and she took several. She subscribed to a newsletter that both evaluated and then sold various vitamin combinations. Currently she took a very potent anti-oxidant mix as well as some specific anti-oxidant pills in high dose, such as Vitamin E, C, and D. She also took folic acid, fish oil, Coenzyme Q-10, and an eye vitamin.

"You can't just take fish oil," she told me. "It has to be the correct omega-3 combination." She turned to a page in one of her newsletters in which an article, written by a doctor wearing a crisp white coat, explained the benefits of his particular formulation of omega 3 fatty acids.

On various occasions we talked about her vitamins. I questioned the need for several of them, and the potential harm they could induce. I rarely had any data to back up my positions, while she had the newsletter to back up hers. "At worst," she told me, "I will fight off colds. At best, I will live longer." She gloated that she had not been sick for years.

On this visit we talked about why she was taking certain of her vitamins. She had no eye disease, but took eye vitamins (a mix of antioxidants in a pill called Preservision™) as a preventive strategy. She had high cholesterol and a family history of heart disease, so she took strong anti-oxidants and fish oil as well as CoQ-10. I was most concerned about vitamin E, since a recent study had shown some danger of high doses of E she now took in her multiple vitamin mixes. I showed her the data. She was skeptical of any studies that looked at vitamins, as she felt they were sponsored by drug companies that intentionally sought to discredit natural remedies.

I also showed her the data on her eye vitamins, explaining that in people without existing macular degeneration, such vitamins had no impact on vision. In fact, Mrs. W still smoked just a few cigarettes, and I explained that one of the ingredients in her eye vitamin (beta-carotene) could increase the risk of cancer in smokers.

After our talk, Mrs. W seemed skeptical about my doubts regarding her many vitamins. But in subsequent meetings, I noticed that her use of supplements diminished.

© Springer International Publishing Switzerland 2015
E. Rifkin, A. Lazris, *Interpreting Health Benefits and Risks*,
DOI 10.1007/978-3-319-11544-3_22

While she continued to show me her newsletter, she started asking whether certain vitamins may be helpful. Within a year, she now only took a few supplements, and they seemed to change from visit to visit. She also quit smoking. As new studies emerged on supplements, I shared them with Mrs. W, and she was appreciative.

A. Key Questions

- Are certain vitamin combinations better than others? Is there a use for multi-vitamins?
- Are there specific vitamins and minerals that may improve a patient's clinical condition? Are there certain vitamins that may be harmful?
- What is the impact of vitamin combinations on a patient's health?
- Is there a proven clinical benefit to any vitamins?

B. Risks and Benefits

- Most vitamins are not well regulated and vary in both composition and dosage. There are very few large, rigorous studies that evaluate the clinical benefit of vitamins on meaningful outcome.
- Multi-vitamins have been shown to have no significant improvement in health outcome, although there is a trend toward benefit. This is true of anti-oxidant combinations as well (Fig. 22.1).
- There is some utility in specific eye vitamins for people with macular degeneration, with a 60/1,000 reduction in progression of visual loss.
- Vitamin E supplementation shows a small increase in overall death (4/1,000) and cardiac events (9/1,000) compared to placebo, with variable results in cancer. A recent small study showed some degree of improvement in function of Alzheimer's patients.
- Folic acid theoretically can reduce homocysteine, which is felt to be a marker for heart disease, but there is no improvement in outcome in people with high homocysteine who take folic acid compared to those who take placebo, and there may be an increased mortality for those who take folic acid and have very high baseline homocysteine levels.
- **Fish oil has shown a trend toward improved cardiac outcome, although no definitive reduction in death or cardiac events. There seems to be an increase of prostate cancer of 24/1,000 in men who take fish oil when compared to placebo (Fig. 22.2).**
- Multiple other vitamins and supplements have too little data to be properly evaluated.

BRCTs:
Vitamins and Supplements

Effectiveness of Multivitamins in Keeping People Healthy

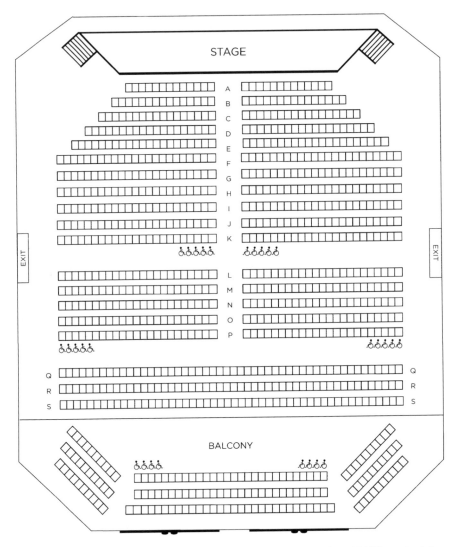

Fig. 22.1 Effectiveness of Multivitamins in Keeping People Healthy. Out of 1,000 people sitting in a theater who use multi-vitamins regularly, none of them, represented by no blackened seats, will improve statistically in terms of any major outcome including reduced death rate compared to 1,000 people who do not take vitamins

Risks of Taking Fish Oil Supplements

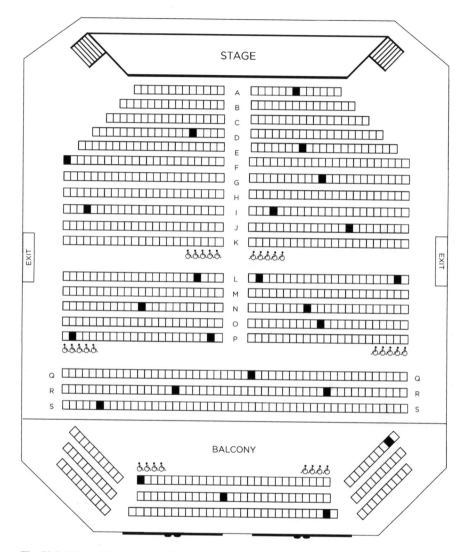

Fig. 22.2 Risks of Taking Fish Oil Supplements. Out of 1,000 men in a theater who take regular fish oil, 24 more, represented by blacked seats, will develop prostate cancer than among 1,000 men not taking fish oil

C. Discussion

Vitamins and supplements are used both as preventive and therapeutic agents. They are available without a prescription, both in stores and on the internet. Most vitamins are not tightly regulated by the FDA. In fact, claims made by vitamin companies can be misleading, and even the contents of certain vitamins and supplements can vary widely from company to company and from pill to pill. Vitamins are not subjected to as many rigorous studies as are prescription medications, and thus our data as to their efficacy and potential side effects are limited.

According to the US Preventive Services Task Force website: "The USPSTF concludes that the evidence is insufficient to recommend for or against the use of supplements of **vitamins** A, C, or E; multivitamins with folic acid; or antioxidant combinations for the prevention of cancer or cardiovascular disease."[1] The site has also explored other specific supplements and reached similar conclusions. We will examine the available evidence for certain vitamins.

Multivitamins come in many forms. They are essentially a mix of many types of vitamins, supplements, and minerals. Some are marketed to provide general nutrition, others for specific purposes (memory improvement, eye health, heart health, etc.). Most multivitamins found in stores contain relatively low doses of their active ingredients, while some of the more potent combinations can be purchased through newsletters or on the internet. Some combination pills are touted to be anti-oxidants, essentially implying that they have strong anti-inflammatory properties that can fight both cancer and vascular disease.

There are many specific anti-inflammatory vitamins that have been studied more extensively, including Vitamin E and Folic Acid, the latter being a B vitamin. Both have theoretical benefits. Vitamin E clears free radicals from tissue, and as a fat soluble vitamin it can penetrate blood vessel tissue. It also blocks platelet function and thus could prevent clot. The latter effect can cause increased bleeding risk, especially when combined with other anti-platelet agents such as aspirin or even fish oil. The maximum safe dose is stated to be 1,500 iu a day. Folic Acid can reduce a chemical in the body called homocysteine. People with high homocysteine levels are more prone to heart attacks and strokes, and thus reducing that level could theoretically mitigate that risk. Folic Acid is a water soluble vitamin that will not accumulate in the body like Vitamin E.

Fish Oil, an Omega-3 Fatty Acid, has been variably shown to help prevent heart attack risk and to perhaps prolong life. The effects of omega-3 fats are to decrease triglycerides, decrease platelet aggregation, and decrease inflammation.

Several other vitamins and supplements have more specific uses. Vitamin C and Echinacea are thought to reduce both severity and duration of upper respiratory infections. Some people take Vitamin C also to prevent colds. Cinnamon, cardamom, and even turmeric are thought to lower blood sugars and perhaps improve memory. Ginko Baloba and even coconut oil are thought to improve memory. Most

---

[1] http://www.uspreventiveservicestaskforce.org/uspstf/uspsvita.htm.

of these have not been well studied, although clinical observations flood both the common press and the internet.

In addition to there being specious data about individual vitamins, there is virtually no available information about the impact of multiple supplements taken simultaneously. For a patient such as Mrs. W, who is taking many individual and combined vitamins and supplement pills, the cumulative effect of her cocktail cannot be ascertained.

Vitamin E: Several studies have examined the risks and benefits of Vitamin E at various doses. Many multi-vitamin combinations have 400 iu of E, while patients can take up to 2,000 iu in individual doses. According the USPSTF, while several cohort studies have shown minor improvement in cardiovascular outcome with vitamin E supplementation, rigorous clinical trials have not.

The HOPE-TOO trial looked at low dose vitamin E in patients with pre-existing vascular disease or diabetes. In this study, 10,000 patients were followed for 7 years. In the E group there was a 7/1,000 decrease in cancer, a 4/1,000 decrease in cancer death, and a 9/1000 *increase* in cardiac events in patients who took E instead of placebo. People on larger doses of Vitamin E had a higher rate of heart failure and hospitalization for heart failure [1]. Another study looked at total mortality with long-term Vitamin E supplementation at various doses. Overall those who took larger doses of Vitamin E had a higher death rate than placebo, with the overall excess rate of death being 3.9/1,000 for people who took E at any dose [2].

Vitamin E has other effects that have been studied. Recently a study demonstrated that men who take vitamin E may have a higher prostate cancer risk. In a mean follow-up of 7-12 years, there was an excess of 1.6/1,000 prostate cancers in men taking Vitamin E vs. placebo [3]. Vitamin E also can potentially help memory, although that impact has been poorly documented in past studies. A 2014 JAMA study that looked at 614 men with Alzheimer's disease who took high dose (2,000 iu) of Vitamin E found a measurable (190/1,000) improvement in their ability to maintain functional activity level over six months. The study had a high drop-out rate which resulted in a very low numbers of patients [4]. The dose used has also been shown to induce an increased risk of bleeding and death in prior studies. Groups like the Alzheimer's Association have called for caution and more study before recommending use of Vitamin E in dementia.

Folic Acid: Many studies have examined the role of folic acid in reducing the level of homocysteine and cardiac death. Two large, recent meta-analyses showed no significant impact of folic acid on cardiac risk, cardiac death, and overall mortality. In one study, those people with the highest baseline homocysteine level actually had worse outcome with folic acid than with placebo [5]. The other analysis looked at 37,500 people through 8 studies over 2.7 years and found 76/1,000 vascular deaths in both groups, 28/1,000 cancer deaths in both groups, and an overall mortality advantage of 2/1,000 favoring placebo [6]. In a longer randomized trial of 5,400 women with high risk of vascular disease studied over 7 years, cardiovascular disease, cardiovascular death, and total death were essentially equal between both groups [7].

Fish Oil: The outcomes of fish oil studies have varied over the years, with most studies showing a trend toward benefit of vascular outcome. Several recent large studies found similar results, without any statistically significant benefit from omega-3 supplementation when compared to placebo. A study of people with known CAD found no change in mortality, heart disease, or stroke in patients who took fish oil vs. those who did not [8]. A study of 12,500 people at high risk for vascular disease showed a 2/1,000 reduction in cardiac death and hospital admission over 5 years in patients who took fish oil, a finding without statistical significance [9]. In a meta-analysis of 20 studies involving 70,000 people there were trends toward improvement with fish oil, and a 4/1,000 improvement in total mortality over 2–6 years, but again nothing reached statistical significance [10].

Fish oil does have potential side effects, some of which are not well documented regarding their prevalence in absolute risk terms. There is a higher bleeding risk, especially when combined with other anti-platelet agents. There also may be a higher prostate cancer risk in men, including a risk of high grade cancers. In a breakdown of SELECT data of 35,000 patients, 24/1,000 patients developed prostate cancer and 4.5/1,000 developed high grade prostate cancer in people who took fish oil vs placebo. There was no indication of how fish oil impacted prostate cancer death [11].

Multi-vitamins: Recent issues of <u>Annals of Internal Medicine</u> published three large trials of multi-vitamins and an editorial which stated that: "With respect to multivitamins, the studies published in this issue and previous trials indicate no substantial health benefit. This evidence, combined with biological considerations, suggests that any effect, either beneficial or harmful, is probably small." [12] The largest review followed 3 trials of multivitamins and 24 other vitamin trials in 400,000 people. The study did find a 3/1,000 decrease in mortality between those who took vitamins vs those who did not, but results varied widely between studies, and they did not reach statistical significance [13]. Another large meta-analysis of 50 studies found similar results, although absolute risk values were not published [14]. Two trials specifically looking at anti-oxidant combinations found a small mortality benefit of the vitamins over many years, but without statistical significance [15, 16].

One type of multi-vitamin that has been recommended is a formulation of anti-oxidants that seem to benefit macular degeneration. These vitamins appear useful in people who have moderate macular degeneration in that they slow progression of the disease and retard visual loss. In a study of 3,640 people with moderate macular degeneration ages 55–80 over 5 years, there was an 80/1,000 reduced progression to advanced disease with vitamins vs. placebo, and a 60/1,000 reduced progression to significant visual loss [17]. Several of these vitamins do contain beta-carotene, which in smokers has been found to increase the incidence of lung cancer and lung cancer death by as much as 10/1,000 [18, 19].

Other Vitamins: Coenzyme Q10 is a naturally occurring vitamin that decreases in our bodies as we age, in those who have congestive heart failure, and in various other muscular conditions. The use of statins also reduces the level of CoQ-10.

A few animal and human studies have been done on this vitamin supplement, hypothesizing that raising the level can help everything from heart disease to diabetes to muscular dystrophies to even longevity.[2] Most studies have been negative or inconclusive. A recent double-blind placebo study, not yet published, followed 420 patients for 10 years with severe congestive heart failure. Subjects taking coq10 had significant improvement compared to placebo: there was a 110/1,000 person advantage in preventing major cardiac events, and an 80/1,000 advantage of averting death when compared to placebo. In advance of its publication, there are many in the academic community already criticizing the study design and results, especially in light of prior studies that did not show such benefit.[3]

No studies have demonstrated an improvement in mental acuity in patients with memory loss who take supplements, including Ginko Baloba and multivitamins [20, 21]. Turmeric has been touted as a potential means of improving behavior and memory in Alzheimer's patients based mostly on observational data and rodent studies, and a recent small 3-week study showed some improved behavior, [22] but no large studies have demonstrated any significant impact of turmeric. A small study of cinnamon showed no improvement in glucose control [23].

Smaller studies, and several studies conducted on animals, do demonstrate some improvement with spices on fasting sugars, but this has never been shown in a large study, nor has anyone demonstrated clinical benefit such as would lead to decreased mortality. A large Vitamin C meta-analysis showed variable results of the vitamin on duration and severity of colds, [24] and a study of Echinacea on colds found that those who believed in the power of Echinacea had a reduction of the length of duration and severity of their colds regardless of whether they received placebo or active medicine [25]. Most vitamins now being regularly used have not been subjected to large, rigorous clinical studies, and it is therefore not possible to comment on their efficacy or potential for harm.

References

1. HOPE-TOO Trial Investigators. (2005). Long term vitamin e supplements in patients with vascular disease or diabetes. *Journal of American Medical Association, 2005*(293), 138–147.
2. Miller, E. R., et al. (2005). Meta-analysis: High-dosage vitamin e supplementation may increase all-cause mortality. *Annals of Internal Medicine, 142*(1), 37–46.
3. Klein, E. A., et al. (2011). Vitamin E and the risk of prostate cancer: the selenium and vitamin E cancer prevention trial. *Journal of American Medical Association, 306*, 1549–1555.
4. Searing, L. (2014). A daily dose of vitamin E may slow early Alzheimer's disease. *The Washington Post, 4*(2014), E3.
5. Miller, E. R., et al. (2010). Meta-analysis of folic acid supplementation trials on risk of cardiovascular disease and risk interaction with baseline homocysteine levels. *American Journal of Cardiology, 106*(4), 517–527.

---

[2] http://www.nlm.nih.gov/medlineplus/druginfo/natural/938.html.

[3] http://www.medscape.com/viewarticle/805099.

6. Clark, R., et al. (2010). Effects of lowering homocysteine levels with b vitamins on cardiovascular disease, cancer, and cause-specific mortalitymeta-analysis of 8 randomized trials involving 37,485 individuals. *Archives of Internal Medicine, 170*(18), 1622–1631.
7. Albert, C. M., et al. (2008). Effect of folic acid and B vitamins on risk of cardiovascular events and total mortality among females at high risk for cardiovascular disease. *Journal of American Medical Association, 2008*(299), 2027–2031.
8. Kwak, S., et al. (2012). Efficacy of omega-3 fatty acid supplements in the secondary prevention of cardiovascular disease. *Archives of Internal Medicine, 175*(9), 686–694.
9. Risk and Prevention Study Collaborative Group. (2013). N-3 fatty acids in patients with multiple cardiovascular risk factors. *New England Journal of Medicine, 368*, 1800–1808.
10. Rizos, E., et al. (2012). Association between omega-3 fatty acid supplementation and risk of major cardiovascular disease events: A systematic review and meta-analysis. *Journal of American Medical Association, 308*(10), 1024–1033.
11. Brasky, T. M., et al. (2013). Plasma phospholipid fatty acids and prostate cancer risk in the SELECT trial. *Journal of the National Cancer Institute, 105*(15), 1132–1141.
12. Gellar, E., et al. (2013). Enough is enough: Stop wasting money on vitamin and mineral supplements. *Annals of Internal Medicine, 159*(12), 850–851.
13. Fortmann, S., et al. (2013). Vitamin and mineral supplements in the primary prevention of cardiovascular disease and cancer: An updated systematic evidence review for the U.S. preventive services task force. *Annals of Internal Medicine, 159*(12), 824–834.
14. Myung, S., et al. (2013). Efficacy of vitamin and antioxidant supplements in prevention of cardiovascular disease: systematic review and meta-analysis of randomised controlled trials. *British Medical Journal, 346*, f10.
15. Bjelakovic, G., et al. (2007). Mortality in randomized trials of antioxidant supplements for primary and secondary prevention. *Journal of American Medical Association, 2007*(297), 842–857.
16. Bjelakovic, G., et al. (2013). Antioxidant supplements to prevent mortality. *Journal of American Medical Association, 310*, 1178–1179.
17. Group, A.-R. E. D. S. R. (2001). A randomized, placebo-controlled, clinical trial of high-dose supplementation with vitamins c and e, beta carotene, and zinc for age-related macular degeneration and vision loss. *Archives of Ophthalmology, 119*(10), 1417–1436.
18. The alpha-tocopherol, beta carotene cancer prevention study group. (1994). The effect of vitamin e and beta carotene on the incidence of lung cancer and other cancers in male smokers. *New England Journal of Medicine, 330*(15), 1029–1035.
19. Omenn, G., et al. (1996). Risk factors for lung cancer and for intervention effects in CARET, the beta-carotene and retinol efficacy trial. *Journal of the National Cancer Institute, 1996*(88), 1550–1559.
20. Snitz, B. E., et al. (2009). Ginkgo Biloba for preventing cognitive decline in older adults. *Journal of the American Medical Association, 302*, 2663.
21. Grodstein, F., et al. (2013). Long-term multivitamin supplementation and cognitive function in men: A randomized trial. *Annals of Internal Medicine, 159*(12), 806–814.
22. Hishikawa, N., et al. (2012). Effect of tumeric on Alzheimer's disease with behavior and psychological symptoms of dementia. *An International Quarterly Journal of Research in Ayurveda, 33*(4), 499–504.
23. Baker, W., et al. (2008). Effect of cinnamon on glucose control and lipid parameters. *Diabetes Care, 3*(1), 41–43.
24. Hemila, H., et al. (2013). Vitamin C for preventing and treating the common cold. *Cochrane Database of Systematic Review, 1*, CD000253.
25. Barrett, B., et al. (2011). Placebo effects and the common cold: A randomized controlled trial. *Annals of Family Medicine, 2011*(9), 312–327.

Chapter 23
MRI and Back Pain

Mr. L came in with back pain. The pain initially grabbed him across the lower spine, keeping him out of work for a week. But now it was even worse. Pain radiated down the right leg, and movement seemed to agitate it. He spent time lying on the floor. He tried taking large doses of Tylenol™ and Aleve™, but those barely took the edge off. He had no other symptoms such as weight loss or fevers. He was a generally healthy 55-year-old man without a significant past medical history other than occasional pangs of back pain throughout his life, although none nearly this severe. Nothing seemed to have instigated this bout of pain; it just emerged one morning when he woke up.

Mr. L's wife drove him in today and he barely could walk to the exam room. They had two simple requests: pain medicine and an MRI. "We need to know what we are dealing with," Ms. L said to me. "This pain is too incapacitating. We need an MRI."

I asked them what they sought to achieve with an MRI that would impact treatment. They brought up surgery or cortisone shots. They said they wanted to rule out something bad like cancer. They also wanted to know if it was a slipped disc.

I discussed the natural history of back pain, the likelihood of him having a slipped disc, the minimal chance of his having cancer, and various pain regimens that may help his symptoms, including a course of narcotics. I reviewed whether it was likely that an MRI could alter our treatment plan. I also talked about false positive MRIs, and the chance of finding a spinal abnormality that may have nothing to do with his current pain. I then brought up when and if an MRI may be beneficial.

"You're saying to give it more time," Mr. L said to me. "Let's treat the pain and see where we are in a few weeks?"

I nodded. "It's up to you," I said. "But these are the facts, and the likelihood of finding something on an MRI that would change what we do is very slim. And you would have to lie in a tube for 40 min, which may not be very kind to your back."

"Can you tell for sure that it's not cancer?" his wife asked me.

© Springer International Publishing Switzerland 2015
E. Rifkin, A. Lazris, *Interpreting Health Benefits and Risks*,
DOI 10.1007/978-3-319-11544-3_23

"I can't. I told you how common cancer is, so it's up to you if it's worth it now. If the pain continues for another month or so, then we can reconsider. I can tell you that even if it's cancer, giving it another month won't change the overall outcome."

Both of them agreed with the plan. They left with a prescription for pain medicine and an appointment to come back in a month should the pain persist.

A. Key Questions

- Does the patient have a history, symptoms, or exam findings that would necessitate the need for an early diagnosis?
- What is the likelihood of the patient having a serious pathology as a cause of back pain, such as cancer, that may alter the type of treatment offered?
- What is the natural history of lower back pain, and how does MRI help improve outcomes?
- What are MRI findings that may occur in patients with back pain, and do those findings correlate to the cause of the back pain? Do they help guide treatment?
- What is the false positive rate of MRI scans? Is there potential harm of getting those scans?
- How effective are epidural injections and surgery for the treatment of back pain if disc herniation is discovered on MRIs?

B. Risks and Benefits

- The risk of cancer is low in patients with lower back pain (approximately 8/1,000) and virtually all such patients have either a history of breast, prostate, or lung cancer, or have suggestive symptoms such as loss of weight.
- **The vast majority of back pain resolves spontaneously after three months despite its underlying cause, with 730/1,000 people having full recovery. There is no evidence that obtaining an MRI alters the natural course of pain or leads to interventions that improve pain (Fig. 23.1).**
- **A large number of people without any back pain have positive MRI findings such as bulging discs, herniated discs, and spinal stenosis. These numbers in patients over 60 are 900/1,000, 360/1,000, and 210/1,000 respectively. The discovery of spinal disease by MRI in those with back pain, then, does not imply that the pain is caused by what the MRI uncovers. Therefore, there is a very high false positive rate in MRI testing, something that has been shown to lead to unnecessary tests, increased disability, and psychological harm (Fig. 23.2).**
- There is some evidence that epidural injections lead to negative long-term outcome, but that spinal surgery may lead to improved long-term outcome, in those people with chronic pain. There is no data regarding the harm and benefit of invasive intervention in those who have acute back pain.

BRCTs:
MRI and Back Pain

Spine Abnormalities in Healthier Older People Picked up on MRI - Even if they have No Pain

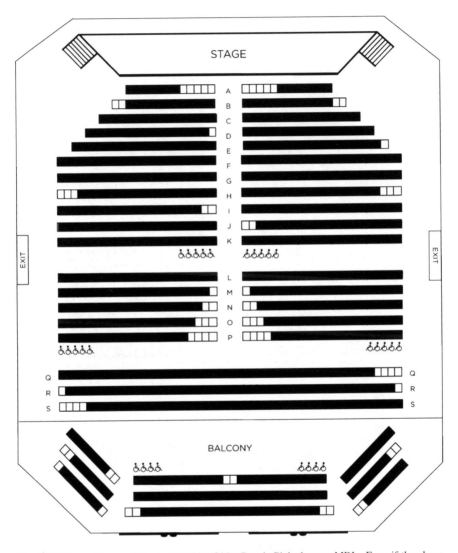

Fig. 23.1 Spine Abnormalities in Healthier Older People Picked up on MRI—Even if they have No Pain. In the general population of people over the age of 60 without any back pain, of 1,000 people in a theater who have MRI scans of their back, 900 people, represented by blackened seats, will have bulging discs, and 360 have herniated discs

Back Pain Improvement Without Treatment

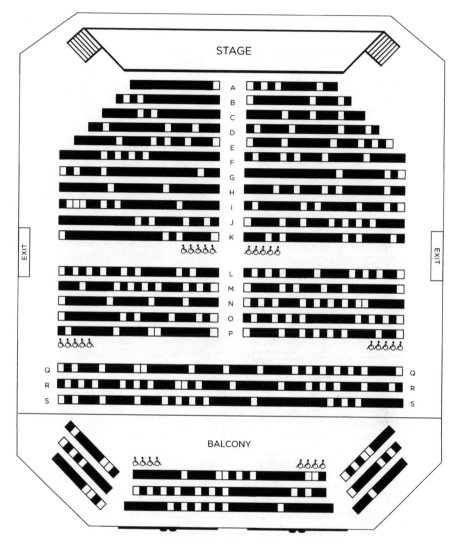

Fig. 23.2 Back Pain Improvement Without Treatment. Out of 1,000 people in a theater with significant back pain, 730, represented by blackened seats, will have full resolution of their symptoms within 3 months whether or not they receive intervention

C. Discussion

Lower back pain is very common, impacting two-thirds of all adults at some point in their lives. Back pain is one of the top ten causes of visits to a doctor's office, and one of the most common causes of disability. Disc herniation, where a disc slips and strikes a nerve, can cause back pain that travels down the leg. Muscle spasm is another prevalent trigger of pain. Metastatic cancer is much less common, although it is what most people fear. It has been found that 7–8/1,000 cases of severe back pain are caused by cancer, and these are typically in people with a history of either breast, lung, or prostate cancer and who exhibit other symptoms such as weight loss. Typically, if metastatic cancer is discovered, it is not curable. Most back pain is never definitively diagnosed, with 850/1,000 cases having no known cause. Also, most back pain resolves spontaneously without the need for specific treatment [1].

MRI is a precise means of looking at the bones, nerves, and discs in a spine. It is common for physicians to order MRIs in patients who present with back pain. In a recent study, the number of MRIs for back pain increased from 72/1,000 in 1999 to 110/1,000 in 2010 [2]. Over half of back MRIs have been deemed to be inappropriate by an expert panel.[1] As to how an MRI can help make a diagnosis, guide treatment, and improve outcome has been studied, and the results of those studies may help patients and doctors decide when and if an MRI is useful for patients such as Mr. L.

The American College of Physicians (ACP) delineated a clinical guideline strongly discouraging the use of MRI in the diagnosis of acute back pain. According to the statement: "Diagnostic imaging is indicated for patients with low back pain only if they have severe progressive neurologic deficits or signs or symptoms that suggest a serious or specific underlying condition. In other patients, evidence indicates that routine imaging is not associated with clinically meaningful benefits but can lead to harms." [3] The study cites the fact that no evidence demonstrates that MRI screening alters outcome or confers any clinical benefit such as improved pain or function.

It also notes that people with back pain who are found to have abnormalities from MRI screening have more stress, are more likely to avoid exercise, and tend to focus on minor symptoms that are not clinically important, with overall worse psychological health. In one study, of 1,800 people followed with lower back pain, those who received an MRI in the first month had no improvement in pain, function, or psychological well being compared to those who had no scan [4]. Part of that finding relates to the significant improvement in symptoms that occur in the first few months without any intervention. In one study, 580/1,000 people with back pain reported elimination of pain and disability within a month, and 730/1,000 in three months. And, 820/1,000 people were able to return to work within a month [5].

One reason to order an MRI is to rule out cancer. According to the ACP analysis of people with significant lower back pain, 8/1,000 had cancer, and all of those had

---

[1] http://www.medpagetoday.com/PrimaryCare/BackPain/38101.

a past history of cancer or symptoms that were concerning for cancer. In fact, only one out of 2,500 people with lower back pain who were scanned had findings that were unanticipated by the history, and there is no evidence that discovering those abnormalities had any impact on outcome.

Physicians often order MRIs to evaluate patients for disc problems, such as herniation. In fact, many people without any back pain have disc disorders, and thus finding those problems on MRI does not imply that the pain is caused by them. In one study, 640/1,000 people without any back symptoms had disc problems discovered by MRI; typically bulges or protrusions [6]. In an MRI study of asymptomatic people over the age of sixty, none of whom reported any back pain or disability, 900/1,000 had bulging discs, 360/1,000 had herniated discs, and 210/1,000 had spinal stenosis [7].

Other studies have demonstrated a similar discordance between the presence of spinal symptoms and spinal disorders discovered on MRI [8, 9]. Therefore, there is a very high potential for false positives when MRIs are performed early in the course of back pain, given that a large number of abnormal MRI findings exist even in the absence of pain. Because of this, it is felt that MRIs ordered within the first month of pain can reveal clinically insignificant disc disease that is felt to be causing pain, leading to unnecessary interventions and an overall worse outcome, [10] in addition to the psychological harm that we have already discussed. There is no data suggesting any improvement in pain, disability, or function attributed to having an early MRI.

Despite the high likelihood that back pain will resolve with conservative treatment, MRI discovered back problems may instigate invasive treatments, especially after pain has been present for a number of months and becomes chronic. Epidural steroid injections are touted as one method of reducing pain in patients with MRI-discovered spinal disease such as herniation and stenosis. One recent study of epidural injections actually shows *worse* long-term outcome, with 100/1,000 more patients showing improved pain and function after 4 years if they *did not* have shots compared to those who did have shots [11].

In those with chronic back pain, a recent study shows that spinal surgery does confer an advantage over conservative treatment after 8 years, with 100/1,000 more people in the surgery arm reporting improved function and pain, although both groups did show improvement. The surgical patients were strictly selected, and there was a high non-compliance rate among those who did not get surgery [12]. There is no data to support the efficacy of surgical intervention in the early course of back pain.

References

1. Jarvik, J., & Deyo, R. (2002). Diagnostic evaluation of lower back pain with emphasis on imaging. *Annals of Internal Medicine, 37*(7), 586–597.
2. Mafi, J., et al. (2013). Worsening trends in the management and treatment of back pain. *Journal of American Medical Association Internal Medicine, 173*(17), 1573–1581.

3. Chou, R., et al. (2011). Diagnostic imaging for low back pain: advice for high-value health care from the american college of physicians. *Annals of Internal Medicine, 154*(3), 181–189.
4. Chou, R., et al. (2009). Imaging strategies for low-back pain: Systematic review and meta-analysis. *Lancet, 373*, 463–472.
5. Pengel, L. H., et al. (2003). Acute low back pain: Systematic review of its prognosis. *British Medical Journal, 327*, 323.
6. Jensen, M. C., et al. (1994). MRI of the lumbar spine in people without back pain. *New England Journal of Medicine, 331*, 69–78.
7. Boden, S. D., et al. (1990). Abnormal magnetic-resonance scans of the lumbar spine in asymptomatic subjects. A prospective investigation. *Journal of Bone and Joint Surgery (American), 72*, 403–408.
8. El Barzouhi, A., et al. (2013). Magnetic resonance imaging in follow-up assessment of sciatica. *New England Journal of Medicine, 2013*(368), 999–1007.
9. Videman, T., et al. (2003). Associations between back pain history and lumbar MRI findings. *Spine, 28*(6), 582–588.
10. Webster, B. S., & Cifuentes, M. (2010). Relationship of early magnetic resonance imaging for work-related acute low back pain with disability and medical utilization outcomes. *Journal of Occupational and Environmental Medicine, 52*, 900–907.
11. Radcliff, K., et al. (2013). Epidural steroid injections are associated with less improvement in patients with lumbar spinal stenosis: A subgroup analysis of the spine patient outcomes research trial. *Spine, 38*(4), 279–291.
12. Lurie, J., et al. (2014). Surgical versus nonoperative treatment for lumbar disc herniation. *Spine, 39*(1), 3.

Chapter 24
Antibiotics in Sinusitis and Bronchitis

KG came to the office in an acute visit slot. He has another sinus infection. He knew the symptoms: pain in the cheek bones, tiredness, runny nose, thick green discharge. He did not have a fever, but he never seemed to be with these infections. They came several times a year, typically with the change in seasons. Now he has started to cough a bit and had to miss work the past 2 days.

"I always try to wait and see which direction it's going," he told me. "I keep drinking water, take Vitamin C, take my cold pills, and just rest. But this time I can tell, it's not getting better. I need antibiotics."

During his many infections, KG liked to pick his favorite antibiotics. Amoxicillin wasn't quite strong enough. Augmentin™ gave him diarrhea. The Zpack™ always seemed to work well. He was always open to any other suggestions I had. "I don't want to get resistant to them," he said. "Maybe it's better to keep changing them. I don't know what I'd do if they stop working."

In the past I talked to KG about the questionable utility of antibiotics in respiratory infections. Now I showed him some data from a recent study showing that essentially antibiotics did not alter the course of the infection. He looked over the numbers, but saw them differently.

"Looks like more people get better faster with the medicine," he said, pointing. "And besides I'm not like everyone else. I know they work for me. And I can't take a chance missing more work."

In the past, KG tolerated virtually all of the antibiotics, although I did tell him that serious side effects could occur at any time, and drug resistance was possible. But when he asked me how likely those were, I told him that such reactions were very rare. He told me that he would rather take his chances.

Having discussed the pros and cons of treatment, I gave KG another Zpack™.

© Springer International Publishing Switzerland 2015
E. Rifkin, A. Lazris, *Interpreting Health Benefits and Risks*,
DOI 10.1007/978-3-319-11544-3_24

A. Key Questions

- How common are sinus infections and bronchial infections? How many of them are bacterial in which antibiotics would be appropriate?
- Are there symptoms that help distinguish viral from bacterial infections?
- If the patient is requesting an antibiotic, what is the reason for the request? How likely would the patient be to accept leaving the office without an antibiotic?
- Without an antibiotic, how likely will the patient be to improve without complications?
- How likely are antibiotics to help the particular infection with which the patient is presenting?
- What are the potential side effects and complications of taking antibiotics?

B. Risks and Benefits

- Sinus infections and bronchitis are common reasons for visits to doctor's offices. It has been estimated that 20/1,000 sinus infections are bacterial, and 100/1,000 bronchial infections are bacterial.
- The rest are viral infections. Viral infections will not improve with the use of antibiotics.
- The symptoms of viral and bacterial infections are similar and difficult to distinguish clinically.
- For bronchitis, 800–900/1,000 patients are improved by day 7 regardless of whether or not they take antibiotics (see Fig. 24.1).
- Findings from studies show that 800–900/1,000 patients with sinus infections receive antibiotics, and 650/1,000 patients with bronchial infections receive antibiotics. Further, 550/1,000 patients with viral infections believe that their condition is improved with antibiotics, which is likely a placebo effect.
- **For sinus infections after 10 days of treatment, 860/1,000 patients on placebo are better, while 910/1,000 patients on antibiotics feel better. The absolute improvement with antibiotics is 50/1,000 over placebo (Fig. 24.2).**
- **With antibiotics, 100/1,000 more patients have side effects than with placebo (Fig. 24.3).**
- There is a slight reduction in duration of illness with antibiotics in people with bronchitis, felt to be less than a day.

BRCTs:
Antibiotics in Sinusitis and Bronchitis

Bronchitis or Sinusitis - Improvement Without Antibiotics

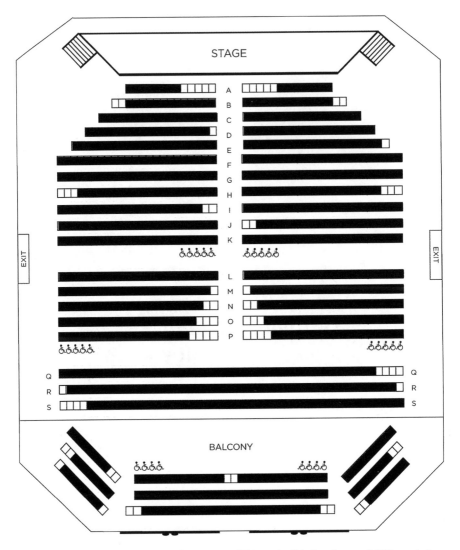

Fig. 24.1 Bronchitis or Sinusitis—Improvement Without Antibiotics. Among 1,000 people in a theater who receive a placebo for sinusitis or bronchitis, approximately 900, represented by blackened seats, will improve by 10–14 days

Antibiotics for Sinusitis or Bronchitis

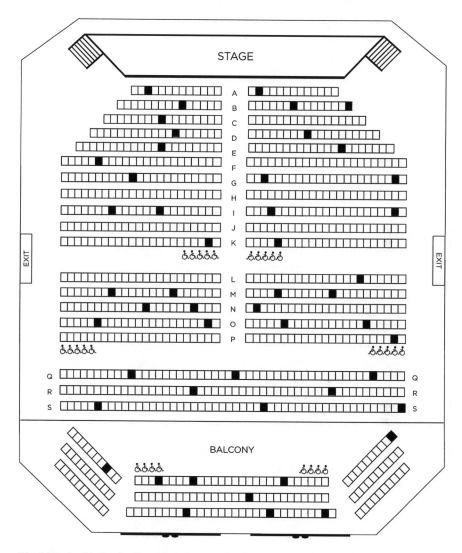

Fig. 24.2 Antibiotics for Sinusitis or Bronchitis. If 1,000 people in a theater take antibiotics for sinusitis, approximately 50 more will improve, represented by blackened seats, than would 1,000 people who take placebo. In bronchitis, there is no statistically significant difference between placebo and antibiotics, and the theater would have no seats darkened

Side Effects from Antibiotics

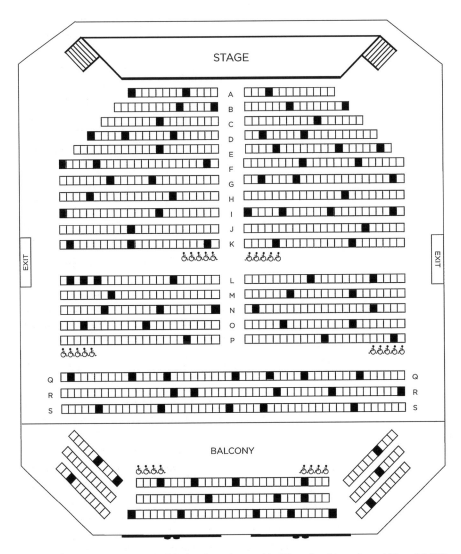

Fig. 24.3 Side Effects from Antibiotics. In patients with either sinusitis or bronchitis, of 1,000 people sitting in a theater who take antibiotics approximately 100, represented by blackened seats, will develop side effects in excess of 1,000 people who take placebo

C. Discussion

Sinusitis is one of the most prevalent conditions prompting patients to visit their doctor and also the primary reason that doctors prescribe antibiotics. Approximately, 30 million Americans are diagnosed with sinusitis annually, and 800–900/1,000 of them received antibiotics from their doctors. It is believed that only 10–20/1,000 of all sinus infections are bacterial, and antibiotics have no impact on non-bacterial, viral infections. But the symptoms and signs of bacterial and viral infections are difficult to distinguish. Nasal congestion, facial pain, runny nose, tooth pain, fever, and fatigue are common to both types of infections. A large ENT society suggests that if symptoms persist more than 7 days and the nasal discharge looks more purulent, then it is more likely that the infection is bacterial. But even then, sinusitis typically resolves spontaneously without any intervention [1, 2].

Many studies explore antibiotic use in acute sinusitis. Most demonstrate some improvement with antibiotic use, although often without statistical significance or large clinical benefit. In several of the studies those on antibiotics do have a trend toward improvement over placebo by the 5th–7th day of treatment, and by day 10 that gap narrows. In fact, both those who use placebo and those given antibiotics show significant improvement by day 10. A Cochrane meta-analysis showed that by day 10–15, 800/1,000 of placebo patients and 900/1,000 of antibiotic treated patients were better. A revision of that analysis in 2014 narrowed the gap between the two groups, with 860/1,000 of placebo patients having improved compared to 910/1,000 of treated patients [3].[1] Therefore, 50/1000 more people on antibiotics improve than those on placebo by day 10.

Both studies also compared the difference between various antibiotics used to treat the sinusitis and found no difference between them. A more recent randomized study comparing amoxicillin to placebo found the 10-day cure rate to be almost identical [4]. Other studies have found varying cure rates, but typically with a small difference between antibiotic and placebo [5].

Study subjects given antibiotics develop side effects in excess of those who use placebo. In the Cochrane meta-analysis, there were 105/1,000 excess side effects in the antibiotic group compared to the placebo group. Most were not severe, and only a small percentage of patients had to drop out of the studies due to side effects. With Augmentin™, though, the side effects were more common and more symptomatic.

Bronchitis is a similarly common diagnosis in primary care, and it often coexists with a sinus infection. Patients with bronchitis typically have a cough, often productive of discolored sputum, with fever, fatigue, and wheezing. Sometimes it is difficult to distinguish bronchitis from more ominous lung infections, such as pneumonia, but typically people with pneumonia are more ill and have distinguishing exam findings. Like with sinusitis, the etiology of bronchitis is viral in 900/1,000 people, and the symptoms of viral and bacterial infection are similar. Still, 650/1,000 of patients presenting with bronchitis receive antibiotics. Many patients are convinced

---

[1] http://summaries.cochrane.org/CD000243/antibiotics-for-acute-maxillary-sinusitis.

that antibiotics are helpful, regardless of their infection's source. In one analysis, 550/1,000 of people who received antibiotics for a viral infection believed that the medicines helped them [6, 7]. Therefore, there is a very strong placebo effect of antibiotic use in respiratory infections.

The antibiotic treatment of bronchitis delivers similar efficacy to that of sinusitis. In a randomized, blinded study of 230 people, patients were given Azithromycin or low dose Vitamin C for bronchitis. Most study subjects exhibited symptoms consistent with bacterial infection including purulent cough and fever. In both groups 890/1,000 of patients recovered by day 7 without any difference in side effects [8]. In a recent study, 461 patients with bronchitis were randomized to Augmentin™, Ibuprofen, or placebo. Results were that 780/1,000 patients on Augmentin™ improved compared to 860/1,000 on Ibuprofen and 860/1,000 on placebo. Also, 120/1,000 of patients developed side effects on Augmentin™, compared to 50/1,000 on Ibuprofen and 30/1,000 on Placebo [9]. Two large meta-analyses found that in general antibiotics reduced the duration of bronchitis symptoms by about a half of a day [10, 11]. Overall, then, there is inconsistency between the studies, with some demonstrating better results with antibiotics, others with placebo, and others showed equal efficacy. In all of the studies, both groups did well with or without treatment, and the difference between the two groups was very small.

References

1. Ah-See, K., & Evans, A. (2007). Sinusitis and its management. *British Medical Journal, 334*, 358.
2. Boisselle, C., & Rowland, K. (2012). Rethinking antibiotics for sinusitis—Again. *The Journal of Family Practice, 61*(12), 610–12.
3. Ahovuo-Saloranta, A., et al. (2008). Antibiotics of acute sinusitis. *Cochrane Database System Review 16*(2)
4. Garbutt, M., et al. (2012). Amoxicillin for acute rhinosinusitis: A randomized controlled trial. *Journal of American Medical Association, 307*(7), 685–92.
5. Williamson, I., et al. (2007). Antibiotics and topical nasal steroids for treatment of acute maxillary sinustis. *Journal of American Medical Association, 298*(21), 2487–96.
6. Albert, R. (2010). Diagnosis and treatment of acute bronchitis. *Am Fam Physician, 82*(11), 1345–50.
7. Wenzel, R., & Fowler, A. (2006). Acute bronchitis. *New England Journal of Medicine, 355*(20), 2125–30.
8. Evans, A. T., et al. (2002). Azithromycin for acute bronchitis: a randomized double blind controlled trial. *Lancet, 359*(9318), 1648–54.
9. Llor, C., et al. (2013). Efficacy of anti-inflammatory or antibiotic treatment in patients with non-complicated acute bronchitis and discoloured sputum: Randomised placebo controlled trial. *British Medical Journal, 347*, f5762.
10. Smucny, J., et al. (2004). Antibiotics for acute bronchitis. *Cochrane Database of Systematic Reviews, 2004*, 4.
11. Bent, S., et al. (1999). Antibiotics for acute bronchitis, a meta-analysis. *American Journal of Medicine, 107*(1), 62–7.

Chapter 25
Final Thoughts

When we decided to write *Interpreting Health Benefits and Risks: A Practical Guide to Facilitate Doctor-Patient Communication* about a year ago, it seemed to us that there was a noticeable commitment within the medical community and among patients to move the concept of shared decision making to a practical level. We reviewed articles, books, and videos which presented a compelling case to move ahead and begin to implement meaningful projects designed to empower patients. Empowerment in this context refers to patients participating in medical discussions and decision making based on the pros and cons of medical intervention that is presented to them in a meaningful and easily understood format.

It is clear that increasingly more doctors and patients are becoming advocates for involving patients in the medical decision making process. At the same time, there are also many barriers to shared decision making including:

- Poorly designed decision aids;
- Patient resistance to changing the status quo whereby doctors tell them what to do;
- Physician resistance to implementing new systems that could be time consuming and may present logistical difficulties; such as the inability to quickly find applicable data;
- Patient inability to understand health risk and benefits;
- Our reliance on relative risks and benefits, which can distort medical information; and
- The financial consequences of advocating for the elimination of over-treatment.

Unfortunately, these warnings and concerns appear to have raised the level of inertia to the point where the discussion now focuses on the potential pitfalls of shared decision making rather than on proposing concrete solutions.

Physicians, patients, pharmaceutical companies, academia, medical journals, the press, other media outlets, government agencies, and insurance companies are, for a variety of reasons, actively involved in discussions related to empowering patients. But discussions and awareness do not necessarily translate into results.

© Springer International Publishing Switzerland 2015
E. Rifkin, A. Lazris, *Interpreting Health Benefits and Risks*,
DOI 10.1007/978-3-319-11544-3_25

Little has been done to provide facile methods to enable meaningful doctor–patient discussions about practical medical issues in an office visit.

For example, representatives from all of the abovementioned groups are well aware of why relative numbers should never be used to characterize health benefits and risks associated with medical intervention. All of these groups understand why the use of relative risk-benefit to inform patients is, to all intents and purposes, misleading, deceptive, and inappropriate. But, this high level of awareness has done little to change the status quo. Medical journals largely still publish their findings using relative numbers, and the press presents new medical information the same way, as do pharmaceutical advertisements about their newest medicines. As long as relative risk-benefit remains the primary language of health care, then useful conversations about medical decisions will be difficult.

Perhaps we are spending too much time arguing about the definition of terms such as shared decision making, patient empowerment, and evidence-based medicine. Maybe the inherent glacial processes associated with solving complex problems and large governmental and bureaucratic agencies have become overwhelming. If true, that would be unfortunate given how the ACA has raised awareness of the patient's role in medical decision making and yet it has done little to facilitate that role.

Perhaps, as we have surmised, the process does not have to be so difficult. By changing the language of medical decision making into one that is meaningful and simple to understand (absolute risk and benefit), and by providing easily presented and digested devices to convey medical information from doctor to patient, patient empowerment can occur without infringing on physician time or interfering with the doctor–patient relationship. In fact, just the opposite will likely occur.

Given all the comprehensive, well-written books published on the subjects of shared decision making and risk-benefit analysis, all espousing the virtues of using absolute risks, is it not time to alter the language of medical communication and establish tools to improve that communication? Currently, in our view, rather than recommending a "path forward" that would pragmatically improve shared decision making, peer-reviewed articles and books on the subject have focused on the need to do something better *without defining what that would be.*

Essentially, *Interpreting Health Benefits and Risks: A Practical Guide to Facilitate Doctor-Patient Communication* is about changing the direction back to—Let's try something concrete! Let's try to actually change the status quo! We believe the use of BRCTs may be of considerable value in achieving the goal of meaningful shared decision making since:

- *We know it works!* One of us is a practicing Internist and has successfully used BRCTs to empower his patients to make decisions on a wide range of medical interventions, many of which are presented in our case studies;
- BRCTs are easy to understand. There is no math, no statistics, no medical jargon, and no complicated charts.
- We have found that presenting information using BRCTs is not time consuming and having patients actively participate is very rewarding for both physician and patient;

- The research used to generate the "blackened dots" in the BRCT is current and consists of findings in robust, unbiased studies;
- The BRCTs present absolute values. They can also be used to illustrate why the use of relative values, to all intents and purposes, will always result in misinformation and confusion;
- Medical journals and other peer-reviewed journals should be able to see the benefits in requiring authors to include BRCTs along with results presented as relative risks. That should enable the press and patients to see, up front, the true meaning of medical data and how individuals are impacted;
- Risks and benefits associated with any kind of medical intervention can be presented on a one page graphic display—the beauty of this approach is in its simplicity;
- BRCTs can be prepared for any form of medical intervention, if the data are available. For example, we could have included BRCTs on cervical cancer screening, shingles vaccines, HPV vaccine, HPV screening, Tamiflu, influenza vaccine, to name a few. If risks and benefits cannot be calculated due to insufficient information, that knowledge should be provided to doctors and patients.

We believe this approach can supplement existing efforts to implement shared decision making. It will raise the level of interest in developing more effective and meaningful decision aids and lead to a universal paradigm with agreed upon criteria. We also are of the opinion that if a few medical journals and a few prominent newspapers agreed to require health risk and benefit information to be presented in absolute values, it would significantly increase the number of empowered patients. We also strongly believe the medical community will benefit from and support this effort. We hope that our book opens the door to a concerted effort that will make shared decisions the norm in most medical practices.

ERRATUM TO

Screening for Carotid Disease in Asymptomatic Patients

© Springer International Publishing Switzerland 2015
E. Rifkin, A. Lazris, *Interpreting Health Benefits and Risks*,
DOI 10.1007/978-3-319-11544-3_14

DOI 10.1007/978-3-319-11544-3_26

The title of chapter 14 was captured incorrectly. The correct chapter title should read:
Screening for Carotid Disease in Asymptomatic Patients.

Also, please ignore the heading **Patients** following the chapter title.

The online version of the original chapter can be found at
http://dx.doi.org/10.1007/978-3-319-11544-3_14

© Springer International Publishing Switzerland 2015
E. Rifkin, A. Lazris, *Interpreting Health Benefits and Risks*,
DOI 10.1007/978-3-319-11544-3_26

Index

A

Abdominal aneurysms, 149
Abnormal stress tests, 11, 84, 85, 88
Absolute benefits, 16, 29, 60, 134, 143,
    144, 180
Absolute risks, 16, 18, 22–24, 26, 39, 44, 48,
    52, 61, 96, 102, 127, 134, 180, 194,
    195, 199, 210, 230
Absolute values, 14–16, 18, 30, 231
ACA. *See* Affordable Care Act (ACA)
Acceptable individual risks, 19, 61
Acceptable risk, 5, 6, 10, 14, 16, 19, 27, 28,
    126, 131, 132, 144
Acute ischemic strokes, 111
ADAS score, 169
Affordable Care Act (ACA), 6, 7, 21, 25, 230
Alendronate, 174, 180
Alzheimer's disease, 10, 168, 169, 209
American Cancer Society, 5, 19, 28, 58, 156
Aneurysm, 149, 155–157
    screening, 155–157
Angiogram, 90–93, 116, 121, 122
Annual exam, 6, 16, 147–158, 173
Annual routine blood tests, 155
Antibiotics, 43, 221–228
Anticoagulation, 97, 101, 103
Anti-inflammatory agent, 111
Anti-oxidants, 203, 204, 208, 210
Anti-platelet agents, 97, 101, 107, 112, 208, 210
Aricept, 161, 169, 170
Aspirin, 96, 97, 99–103, 105–112, 208
Asymptomatic, 11, 44, 46–48, 59, 84, 87,
    91–93, 115–122, 155, 157, 161,
    179, 219
Atherosclerosis, 122, 127, 130, 132141
Atrial fibrillation, 95–103, 155

B

Back pain, 179, 213–219
Bacterial infections, 222, 227, 228
Benefit/Risk Characterization Theaters
    (BRCT), 14–16, 18, 19, 22–30, 45–49,
    66–72, 74, 76–81, 86–93, 98–103,
    108–112, 117–122, 128–132, 136–144,
    150–158, 164–170, 176–181, 185–191,
    196–200, 205–211, 215–219, 223–228,
    230, 231
Benign prostate hyperplasia
    (BPH), 47
Biomarker, 58
Biopsy, 3–5, 33, 34, 37, 51, 52, 58–60, 64, 65,
    70, 71, 158
Bisphosphonate, 25, 174, 175, 177, 178, 180,
    181, 183
Bladder cancer, 81, 149, 156
    screening, 156
Bleeds, 97, 100, 102, 103, 107, 122
Blood serum cholesterol, 14–15, 126, 127,
    129–132, 134, 141, 144
Bone density, 5, 16, 21, 23, 25, 173–181,
    189, 191
    scan, 16
    testing, 173–181
Brain scan, 168
BRCT. *See* Benefit/Risk Characterization
    Theaters (BRCT)
Breast cancer, 17, 24, 25, 27–29, 33–40, 69,
    81, 193–195, 199, 200
    risk, 195
    screening, 27–29, 33–40
Bronchitis, 81, 221–228
Bruits, 149, 157
Bypass surgery, 22, 83, 84, 90, 91

© Springer International Publishing Switzerland 2015
E. Rifkin, A. Lazris, *Interpreting Health Benefits and Risks*,
DOI 10.1007/978-3-319-11544-3

C

Calcitonin, 181
Calcium, 26, 39, 83, 183–191
Cardiac catheterizations, 85, 91, 92
Carotid
    blockage, 116, 121
    disease, 115–122, 149, 157, 158
    stenosis, 121, 157
    ultrasound, 22, 115–120, 147, 157
Carotid artery
    screening, 156–157
    stenosis, 121
Carotid endarterectomy (CEA), 121, 122
Case studies, 19, 27, 30, 230
Castelli, W.P., 131
Cataracts, 81, 135, 139, 141
CHD. *See* Coronary heart disease (CHD)
Chest x-rays, 63, 69, 70
Cholesterol, 5, 14–16, 18, 21, 24, 93, 115,
        125–144, 147, 154, 155, 203
Cholesterol screening, 14, 16, 125–132, 141,
        154, 155
Cholinesterase inhibitors, 162, 169, 170
Chronic health endpoints, 7
CIBC criteria, 169
Clinical guidelines, 5, 6, 21, 112, 218
Clinical practice guidelines, 6, 179
Clopidogrel, 103, 107, 112
Clot, 95, 101, 121, 135, 142, 194, 195, 199, 208
Cochrane collaboration, 9
Coenzyme Q10, 210
Colon cancer deaths, 44, 46, 48, 49
Colon cancer screening, 43–49
Colonoscopy, 6, 14, 17, 43–49
Colon polyps, 44, 48
Communicating health risks and benefits, 7, 17
Comparative-effectiveness research, 7
Comprehensive physical exam, 155
Compression fractures, 175, 179, 181
Congestive heart failure, 97, 101, 210, 211
Controllable risk factor, 130, 142
Coronary heart disease (CHD), 14–16, 18, 74,
        80, 81, 93, 126, 127, 129–132, 134,
        135, 137, 138, 141–144
Coumadin, 95, 96
Crestor, 141
CT scan, 7, 63–65, 67, 68, 70, 71, 83, 90, 161
Cystic breasts, 25
Cystoscopic evaluation, 156

D

DeBakey, M.E., 130
Decision aids, 8–11, 13–19, 27, 30, 229, 231

Dementia, 10, 161–170, 200, 209
Dementia drugs, 10, 162, 163, 166, 167,
        169, 170
Diabetes, 21, 60, 73, 83, 84, 90, 97, 101, 111,
        113, 142, 143, 147, 209, 211
Digital rectal exam (DRE), 51, 58
Disc herniation, 214, 218
Donepezil, 169, 170
DRE. *See* Digital rectal exam (DRE)

E

Echinacea, 208, 211
Echocardiograms, 11, 83, 147
EKGs, 16, 83, 91, 147, 149, 154, 155, 157,
        158, 173
    screening, 157
Elevated cholesterol, 15, 16, 18, 126, 127,
        130–132, 141
Empowering patients, 4, 7, 11, 229
Erectile dysfunction, 52, 59, 61, 81
Estrogen, 23, 24, 181, 193–200
Estrogen replacement therapy,
        193–200
Evidence-based decision, 27
Evidence-based medicine, 7, 230
Evista, 181
Exercise, 22, 63, 73, 74, 83–93, 147, 173,
        193, 218
Exercise stress tests, 22, 83–93

F

Fall prevention, 187
False negatives, 22, 59, 92, 116, 121, 122, 149,
        154–158
False positives, 11, 22, 23, 25, 28, 33,
        34, 37, 40, 48, 51, 59, 63–65,
        68–71, 84, 85, 88, 91–93, 115,
        116, 118, 121, 147–149, 152–158,
        213, 214, 219
False positive x-rays, 69
FDA. *See* Federal Drug Administration
Federal Drug Administration (FDA), 131, 169,
        181, 208
    approved drugs, 169
Fein, D., 92
Femur, 175, 178, 181
Fish oil, 105, 107, 111, 203, 204, 207,
        208, 210
Folic acid, 203, 204, 208, 209
Forteo, 174, 181
Fosamax, 174, 180
Framingham study, 130, 131

G

Genetic mutation, 39
GERD drugs, 179
Ginko Baloba, 208, 211
Graphic, 13, 14, 16, 27, 30, 231

H

Hadler, N, 18, 90
Health effects of smoking, 73–81
Heart attacks, 5, 7, 11, 19, 24, 69, 73, 84, 85,
        88–93, 96, 97, 105, 107, 111, 112, 122,
        125, 126, 130, 131, 133, 134, 137, 138,
        141–144, 183, 184, 190, 200, 208
Hegsted, M., 131
Hemorrhage, 71, 103
High radiation PET scans, 65
Hip fracture, 163, 167, 170, 174, 175, 177,
        179–181, 184, 186, 188–190, 194,
        195, 199
Homocysteine, 204, 208, 209
Hypertension, 73, 83, 84, 97, 122
Hypothyroidism, 155, 168

I

Impotence/impotent, 52, 56, 60, 61
Incontinence/incontinent, 52, 53, 57, 59–61, 199
Individual acceptable risk, 19, 27, 28, 132
Individual risks, 19, 26, 27, 61, 105, 131
Indolent, 52, 59, 60, 71
Ischemic stroke, 96, 97, 101, 102, 111, 112

K

Kannel, W.B., 130
Kidney stones, 184, 189

L

Lipitor, 141–144
Liver dysfunction, 140
Lumpectomy, 39
Lung biopsies, 65, 68, 70, 71
Lung cancer, 7, 19, 63–72, 74, 77, 80, 81, 210,
        214

M

Mammograms, 5, 14, 17, 22, 24, 25, 27–29,
        33–40, 154, 173, 174
Mastectomy, 39
Medical community, 6, 10, 14, 19, 27, 28,
        229, 231

Medical intervention, 4, 5, 7, 9, 11, 13–15,
        17–19, 22, 27, 30, 85, 229–230
Medicare reform, 21
Melanoma, 158
Memantine, 162, 169, 170
Meta-analysis, 112, 155, 168, 170, 190, 191,
        210, 211, 227
Metastasize, 39
Metastatic cancer, 218
Micro-calcifications, 39
Mild cognitive impairment, 169
Moles, 158
Mortality rate, 156, 158
MRI, 161, 213–219
Multiple Risk Factor Intervention Trial
        (MRFIT), 131
Multivitamins, 206, 208, 210, 211
Myopathy, 135, 141

N

Nasal congestion, 227
National Cancer Institute, 53, 58, 60, 158
Nationwide health risks, 131
Non-melanoma skin cancer, 149, 158
Non-osteoporotic T score, 180
Non-vertebral fracture, 181

O

Omega-3 fatty acid, 208
Osteopenic, 180
Osteoporosis, 25, 173–181, 183–191
Overall survival advantage, 71
Over-treatment, 229

P

Palpable lump, 39
Parkinson's dementia, 168
Patient-centered approach, 25–26
Patient preference, 7, 10, 19
Perforations, 43, 44, 47, 49, 156
Placebo, 106, 107, 109, 110, 112, 163, 166,
        167, 169, 170, 177, 178, 180, 184, 186,
        187, 190, 191, 193, 195, 197–198, 204,
        209–211, 222, 224–228
Platelets, 111, 208
Positive stress tests, 22, 84, 85, 92, 93
Post-menopausal, 23, 179, 180, 190,
        198–200
Pravachol, 141, 142
Pre-cancerous polyps, 48
Premarin, 181, 193

Primary prevention, 106, 107, 111, 112, 134,
      137, 142, 143
Progesterone, 24, 193–195, 199, 200
Prostate, 3, 5, 19, 51–61, 69, 149, 153, 155,
      156, 204, 207, 209, 210, 214, 218
Prostate cancer, 3, 5, 51–61, 69, 149, 156, 204,
      207, 209, 210, 218
   screening, 51–61
Prostate cancer outcomes study (PCOS), 60
Prostatectomy, 53, 60
Prostate-specific antigen (PSA), 3, 51, 58
   screening, 53, 58, 60

Q
Quinlan, K.A., 6

R
Radiation, 34, 38–40, 52, 53, 55–57, 63, 65,
      69–71
Rectal bleeding, 48
Rectal cancer, 149, 156
Rectal exam, 16, 51, 58, 149, 153, 156
Relative risk reduction, 17, 18
Relative risks, 14–18, 22–24, 28, 102, 199,
      229–231
Relevant outcomes, 11, 25
Rhabdomyolysis, 134, 141
Rifkin, E., 22
Risk acceptance, 14
Risk aversion, 14
Russert, T., 92

S
Screening for carotid disease, 115–122
Screening tests, 5–7, 11, 14, 19, 21, 22, 27, 30,
      55, 58–60, 63, 91, 130, 149, 154, 156
Secondary prevention, 106, 107, 111, 112,
      134, 138, 142–144
Shared decision making, 3–9, 11, 14, 229–231
Sinusitis, 221–228
Skin screening, 158
Smoking, 3, 26, 63, 65, 69, 73–81, 83, 84,
      121, 142, 154, 179, 204
Spine fracture, 174–175, 179–181, 190
Spiral CT scan, 7, 63, 67, 68, 70, 71
Squamous cell cancer, 158
Statins, 14, 24, 125, 127, 131, 133–144,
      147, 210

Stents, 22, 84, 85, 90, 91, 93
Stress tests, 11, 22, 26, 83–93, 147, 154, 157
Stroke, 5, 24, 69, 73–75, 80, 81, 85, 88, 90,
      91, 93, 95–97, 99–103, 105–112, 115,
      116, 119–122, 125, 130, 147, 148, 157,
      184, 190, 194, 195, 199, 200, 208, 210
Supplements, 21, 23, 24, 102, 105–107, 111,
      147, 183, 184, 188–191, 203–211

T
Thallium, 73, 90, 92
Thrombosis, 111, 142, 181
Thyroid testing, 155
Tumor, 39, 58–60, 168
Turmeric, 208, 211

U
Uncertainty, 5, 7, 23–24, 27, 52, 60, 81, 101,
      142, 168
Universal decision aid, 13–19
Unnecessary treatment, 34, 38, 40
Urinalysis, 156
US Preventative Services Task Force
      (USPSTF), 5, 7, 48, 49, 64, 65, 70, 91,
      111, 112, 121, 122, 155–158, 168, 179,
      180, 189–191, 199, 200, 208, 209
Uterine cancer, 193, 194, 199

V
Valvular heart disease, 101, 155
Vertebral fracture, 181
Viral infections, 222, 227
Vitamins
   vitamin A, 208
   vitamin C, 208, 211, 221, 228
   vitamin D, 183–191
   vitamin E, 23, 105, 107, 203, 204, 208, 209
Vytorin, 141

W
Warfarin, 14, 95–103
Welch, G, 18, 40, 71
Wender, R.C., 28

Z
Zocor, 141–144,